I0047658

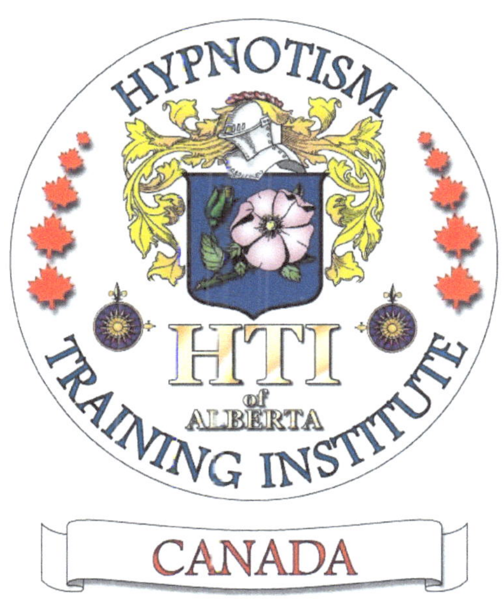

Hypnosis 203

Advanced Clinical Hypnotherapy

By Anny J. Slegten

Advanced Clinical Hypnotherapy
Anny Slegten
Published by
Kimberlite Publishing House
www.kimberlitePublishingHouse.com

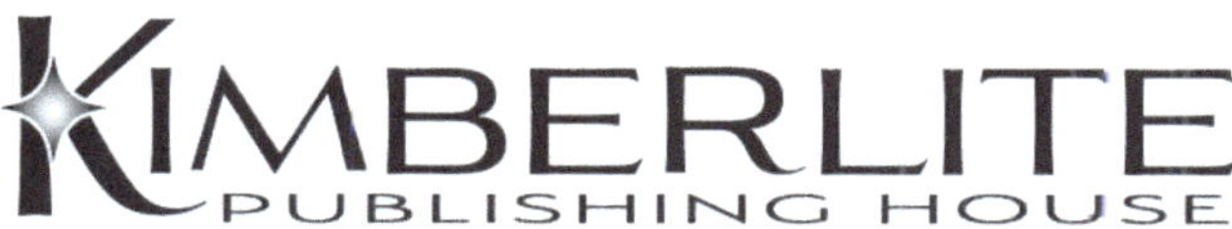

ISBN: 978-1-7752489-7-2

School Coat of Arms designed by Boomer Stralak
Book layout by Colin Christopher *www.colinchristopher.com*
Book cover and Kimberlite Logo designed by Marietta Miller
www.execugraphx.com

The Kimberlite-Diamond Connection

Kimberlite is a rock type that was first categorized over a 100 years ago based on descriptions of the diamond-bearing pipes of Kimberley, South Africa.

Kimberlites are the mechanism by which diamonds are brought to the surface.

Kimberlitic rocks are the most important primary source of diamonds and the main rock type in which significant diamond deposits have been found so far.

Anny is familiar with many rocks and minerals as her husband was raised around quarries, and later worked in several mines in Canada.

Therefore, it was natural for Anny to choose kimberlite as an analogy to the soul residing within our body – as a diamond within the kimberlite.

A Picture Is Worth A Thousand Words – The Swing

Using hypnosis as a technique, you are now entering the second phase of training - Regression Hypnotherapy.

During one-on-one sessions, clients often connect with their inner child. This is the reason I chose a picture of the swing in my yard - it is a perfect image to help you understand what clients experience.

The mind is deductive and goes from effect back to cause. The cause can be anything between a recent situation all the way to a past life.

As you enjoy the training, you will discover that everything has a beginning, and, if your client so desires… everything can be fixed when they go from effect back to cause.

When looking at yourself - you may realize this goes for you too!

Anny

Welcome to

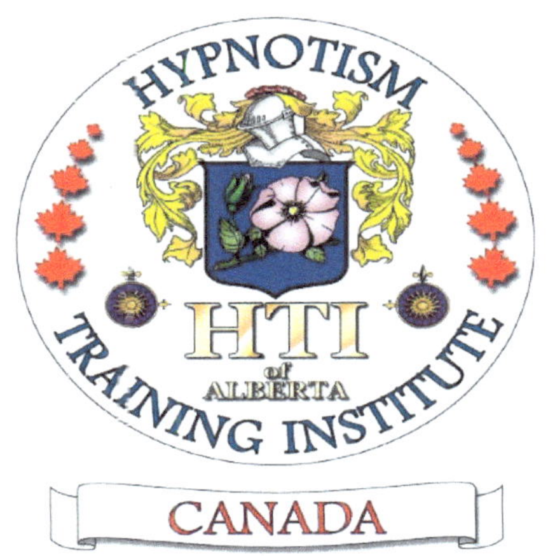

HYP 203 – Advanced Clinical Hypnotherapy

This book belongs to:

Name ______________________________

Mailing Address ______________________________

____

City or Town ______________________________

Province/State ____________________ Postal Code/Zip ________

Country ______________________________

Telephone Home (___) __________ Work (___) __________

Instructor's Name: ***Anny Slegten***

Today's Date: ______________________________

Table Of Contents

A Note From Anny

The design and development of the Course Material required the investment of substantial effort, time, and money.

The transcripts include the actual trance inductions and therefore is to be kept confidential. and is only intended for the participants of HYP 203, Advanced Clinical Hypnotherapy.

Understand that the experiences derived from attending this course is a private and personal experience for each participant. As such please do respect the confidentiality of all participants and their remarks and actions and keep all such information private and confidential.

As a result, I am counting on you do your part at keeping this course environment safe and secure for all participants.

Enjoy!

Your Notes

Anny's Teaching

From A Chicken To An Eagle

According to an old Hindu legend, there was a time when all men were gods, but they so abused their divinity that Brahma, the Chief God, decided to take it away from men and hide it where they would never again find it. Where to hide it became the big question.

When the Lesser Gods were called into council to consider this question, they said" We will bury man's Divinity deep in the earth". But Brahma said, "No, that will not do, for man will dig deep into the earth and find it."

Then they said, "Well, we will sink his Divinity into the deepest ocean." But again, Brahma replied, "No, not there, for man will learn to dive into the deepest waters, will search out the ocean bed and will find it."

Then the Lesser Gods said, "We will take it to the top of the highest mountain and there hide it." But again, Brahma replied "No, for man will eventually climb every mountain on earth. He will be sure some day find it and take it up again for himself."

Then the Lesser Gods gave up and concluded, "We do not know where to hide it for it seems that there is no place on earth or in the sea that man will not eventually reach."

Then Brahma said, "Here is what we will do with man's Divinity. We will hide it deep down inside man himself, for he will never think to look for it there."

Ever since then, the legend concluded, man has been going up and down the earth, climbing, digging, diving, exploring…searching for something that is already within himself.

Author Unknown.

Your Notes

Anny's Teaching

Anchoring

Anchors are the natural associations or associated feelings we make with almost everything in our world. Feelings we experience and connect with such things as people, places, events, and so on.

Anchoring is the technology to be able to deliberately manipulate these many associations. For example, we can disconnect the bad feelings connected to specific memories or situations and conversely, we can connect any powerful great feeling or resource to any stimulus of our choosing such as any person, place, situation. The possibilities are limitless.

Anchors can be created through any sensory channel in two ways.

The first is by repetition. If you repeatedly see a certain look on someone's face when they are in a certain mood, that facial expression will become anchored. This is simple learning. That look means that mood.

Society and everyday living has even installed anchors within us with the colors red as "danger" and green as "go" or "safety".

Secondly, and more importantly, anchors can be set in a single instance if the emotion is strong enough and the timing is right.

Anchoring – Integrating The Two Brains

Basically, anchoring is making an association at a subconscious level. Therefore, it helps a client access a feeling, even when they are hesitating to do so, by merely touching the anchor. It speeds up the sessions, making the client move through unpleasant reviews quickly.

Your Notes

Anny's Teaching

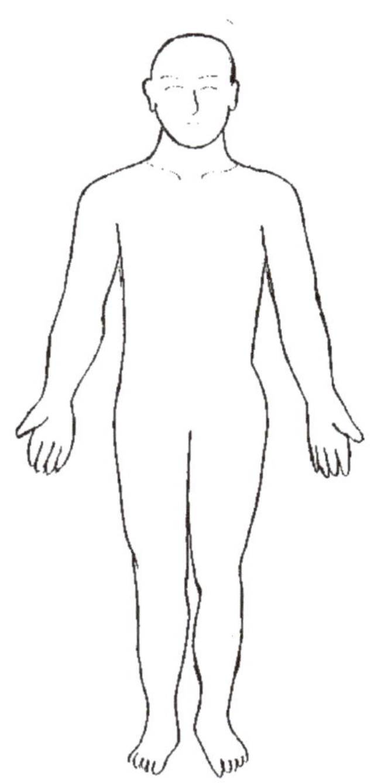

It is the anchor to any person, situation, or event that makes an illusion our reality.

Anchoring the undesirable feelings at the same place on one side of the body and anchoring the desirable feelings on the same place on the other side of the body deals with the two sides of the brain. And when the time is right, when you collapse the anchors by touching and holding the desirable feelings and then touch, let go, touch, let go the undesirable feelings while holding the desirable feelings, you are facilitating the connections and integration of the two sides of the brain. It is like seeing the two sides of a coin simultaneously.

The results: inner peace that comes with self-acceptance. For simplicity, I consistently anchor the undesirable feelings on the left knee and the desirable feelings on the right knee. It quickly becomes automatic, and I can proceed with the hypnotherapy session without having to think about which side is which. Once you have practiced these methods, you will realize how easy they are, by experiencing these methods, you will understand the incredible healing feelings associated with them.

Your Notes

Anny's Teaching

More On Anchoring

Anchoring is an association at subconscious level, and it creates a "trigger"

Example: for my German friend the sound – and smell – of fireworks "triggers" gunfights memories.

That is when A = A = A, as explained in Dianetics.

During a session, we intentionaly anchor some feelings with a touch of a knee. The touch then becomes a "trigger" and the feelings are coming back the moment we touch the knee.

To cancel all the anchors we created to speed up things in a session, at the end make the person talk about and feel a good experience.

And while the person is in the good experience, hold on to the "good: knee as you touch and let go, touch and let go the "bad knee"

And when you feel you did enough of this, STILL HOLDING THE 'GOOD' KNEE, completely let go of the "bad" knee and only then can you let go of the "good" knee.

Thus, having the client experience and be in the "good" feeling, you hold on to the good knee until the very end.

Your Notes

Anny's Teaching

Information – The Church Of Scientology

2009 PARIS - The Church of Scientology could be dissolved in France if it is convicted in a trial that opened Monday in a Paris court, where the group and seven of its French leaders stand charged of organized fraud and illegal pharmaceutical activity.

The group, considered a sect in France, has faced prosecution and difficulties in registering its activities in many countries.

The trial comes more than a decade after one of the three plaintiffs originally filed a complaint against the Church of Scientology. A young woman said she took out loans and spent the equivalent of close to US$30,000 on books, courses and "purification packages" after being recruited by the group in 1998. When she sought reimbursement and to leave the group, its leadership refused.

Investigating judge Jean-Christophe Hullin spent years examining the group's activities, and in his indictment criticized practices he said were aimed at extracting large sums of money from members and plunging them into a "state of subjection."

The investigator questioned what he called the Scientologists' "obsession" with financial gain, and the group's practice of selling vitamins, leading to the charge of "acting illegally as a pharmacy."

Patrick Maisonneuve, lawyer for the Church of Scientology in France, dismissed any organized fraud, although he acknowledged there could have been individual abuses.

"The discovery of a pedophile priest does not allow us to question the entire Catholic Church," he was quoted as saying in the weekly L'Express magazine ahead of the trial opening.

Your Notes

Anny's Teaching

The Los Angeles-based Church of Scientology, founded in 1954 by the late science fiction writer L. Ron Hubbard, has been active for decades in Europe but has struggled to gain status as a religion. The U.S. State Department has criticized Belgium, Germany and other European countries for labeling Scientology a cult or sect and enacting laws to restrict its operations.

A guilty verdict in the current French trial could shut down the group's activities in France.

The investigating judge also questioned the validity of an "electrometer" sold to members for 4,800 euros (about C$7,500) and used to measure variations in their mental state. The judge, in the indictment, called it "an illusion aimed at giving a scientific sense to an operation that has nothing of the kind."

Unusually, the Paris prosecutor's office had recommended the charges be dropped, but the court agreed to take up the case.

In 2002, a French court fined the Paris regional branch of the church for a data protection violation but acquitted it of attempted fraud and judges refused to disband it.

The Church of Scientology teaches that technology can expand the mind and help solve problems. It claims 10 million members around the world, including celebrity devotees Tom Cruise and John Travolta.

Your Notes

Anny's Teaching

Emotional Stress Release

An Emotional Lift

DURING THIS SESSION, MAKE SURE YOU "DOWNLOAD" THE ENERGY THROUGH YOUR FEET.

Highly effective in putting the client back together for clarity of thoughts so the event/issue becomes a story – it becomes a non – issue.

At the end of the session, lightly hold the frontal eminence with one hand and the Primary Visual Areas with the other hand.

- Ask the client to review the session and all the insights gained through the session.

- Ask the client to go to the cause of what was affecting them (Tapping the Primary Visual Areas) and review how it affected them from then all the way to now. (Tapping the frontal eminence).

- When finished, ask the client to rewind the movie of time from now all the way to the beginning at twice the speed it took to review it.

- Repeat several times. Please note: There is no pulse when the client does not process anything, holding on to "it" and stopped breathing.

- Observe the client. Making sure they continue to breathe and going into the process of resolving the emotion attached to the issue,

- When having a clear information, each time the client goes back, I ask my client to go "further back in time", as far back as their mind wants to go, and review everything from then on to now.

- Towards the end of the review, ask the client to allow their mind to go all the way as far back as their mind wants to go, and hold, making sure they breathe through it.

Your Notes

Anny's Teaching

End of the session:

- Ask the person to review the whole thing and to stop at the top of their head to what they perceive is the crucial point in the series of events.

- As the client stops at the significant event, instruct them to review the issue simultaneously from where they stopped back to the beginning and from where they stopped all the way to now at the speed you will move your hands from the frontal/occipital holding to the top of the head and back to the frontal/occipital holding.

- Have the client do this entire exercise until you feel a continuous pulse. Take your time and allow your client to go through this at their own pace. The results are worth it.

- Sometimes, you will feel it is important to have them do the review two to three times and then stop at the top of their head to what they perceive is the crucial point in the series of events.

- When appropriate, get the client to have the residues of the session put in the container, and so forth.

Variation:

Note: Sometimes, once in a trance, the client draws a blank and replies "nothing" to any suggestions. Do, then, the complete exercise, asking the client to go to the beginning of the "nothing" and review the "nothing" from the beginning all the way back to now, etc., The results are the same!

Your Notes

Anny's Teaching

The "Care Package"

Anchoring During The Complete Exercise

Useful to help a person resolve Unfinished Business, getting something off their chest.

It could be a person or a pet to which you were not able to say goodbye to.

It could be a person or a pet still living or dead with whom you still have unresolved feelings.

Note: First ask if the client who hurt them the most, etc. as well as if who they will send this is still living.

Remember to anchor as you read the questions aloud to help the body release the hurt.

In their mind, have a box in front of them. In the privacy of their own mind, in that box, ask them to put.... ....
Each time ending by saying: **"*and when it is done, please say so*"**

- Everything you ever wanted to tell them. How you feel about them. The hurt afflicted. How you feel about the unfinished business. Put in all your thoughts about the unresolved issues. Be explicit and to the point.

- Now, put in the box a picture of you then (the way they remember you), and the way you are now.

- Put in the box pictures or a movie of what upsets you most about them.

Your Notes

Anny's Teaching

- Put in the box pictures or a movie of what you like the most about them
- Then, put in the box pictures or a movie of the saddest time you experienced together.
- Then, put in the box pictures or a movie of the funniest time you experienced together.
- Next, put in the box how you want them to view you. Put in the box how you want them to think of you, respond to you.
- Update them. Let them know how you are now, what you are doing, your personal life, your occupation, your skills, your hobbies, anything else you want to put in that box.
- Put a gift in that box. Something you know they would really like the pleasure to have.
- Fill up the box with your love (when appropriate), your suggestions for their wellbeing, your wishes for them, and lots of laughter.
- Still some room? When appropriate, put flowers in the box too.

Close the box. Gift-wrap it. Put a mailing label on it.
Write on it your name as the sender and for who it is, along with their address.

Decide how that box will be delivered ***and voice it.***
If they are dead, you can call up someone who passed away and cares for you, Angels or Saints or you can carry the box in front of the light and ask them to meet you there.

As a loved one is meeting you there, say your goodbyes. Exchange wishes and recommendations, ask for any advice they have for you.

Your Notes

Anny's Teaching

When still alive, decide who is going to deliver the box: a courier, the postal service, or yourself.

Instruct or decide the time and where the box will de delivered: on the foot of their bed, on the coach, the kitchen table, on their car diver seat, where you are sure the person will be aware of the package and open the box.

And know it is a done deal.

Your Notes

Anny's Teaching

Congruent Integration

Taught in Educational Kinesiology and sometimes called 'Part Therapy".

(Sometimes used as a tool to call the client's bluff)

Highly effective when the client experiences a severe conflict within

At the end of the session, the client still in a trance, put the client's hands apart, palm down. (I lift my client's arms off the recliner's armrests), and say:

"There is a part of you that wants to have the pleasure of ... (breathing easily, for example). That part of you, that wants the pleasure of breathing easily, let it come to one of your hands, and when it is there, turn your hand up so I know you are holding it ..."

When the client signals the "part" has chosen one of the hands, thank the part who wants the pleasure of breathing easily and suggest to the client further saying:

"Deep down, there is a part of you that knows how to have the pleasure of breathing easily. That part of you, that knows how to have the pleasure of breathing easily, let it come into the other hand, and when it is there, turn up your hand so I know you are holding it ..."

When the client signals the other "part" is in the other hand, acknowledge it by saying "thank you".

Now, addressing the client, you say:

Your Notes

Anny's Teaching

"The part of you that wants to have the pleasure of breathing easily and the part of you that knows how to do it, these two parts, there was a time when they were one. They want to be one again. Feel the attraction! It is like powerful magnets in the palm of your hands. Feel the attraction! These two parts, there was a time when they were one.

Let them join again, feel the attraction!

They want to come home ... let them come home ... *observe the hands moving towards each other as you repeat the suggestion, and continue:* Welcome them home, welcome them home ... and when your hands are joining, draw the parts into your heart, welcome them home ... when the integration is completed, and only then, will you be able to open your eyes ... welcome then home, welcome them home."

NOTE: watch for the subconscious movement.

At the end, I say "...and when the integration is completed, only then will you be able to open your eyes, feeling refreshed, relaxed, at peace with yourself and with the world around you...."

The client's feedback is always most interesting.

As you know, there is always variations on the use of any method. One of them is when the client does not consciously acknowledge resistance to their own request.

In that case, the hand, "Who Knows How" **moves toward** the other hand while the hand "That Wants To" **moves away** from the other hand. I ask then the client to open their eyes so they become consciously aware of their inner conflict.

Your Notes

Anny's Teaching

Edu-K Integration Metaphor

This technique was learned at Educational Kinesiology classes using muscle testing.

1. Into one hand, place the parts of you that already has the pleasure to know how to … … (the goal).

2. And into the other hand, place the parts of you that have not yet had the pleasure to learn … … (the goal).

3. I respectfully ask the subconscious mind to do whatever is needed to have the pleasure of making … … (the goal) a congruent belief for system.

Allow your hands to come together whenever you are ready.
When joined, bring them into your body.

Muscle test: Is the integration completed?

Note:

During an Ericksonian Hypnosis course taken in February 1997, Dr Rossi, using the same idea, asked:

"WHAT DO YOU HAVE IN THE OTHER HAND BY CONTRAST?"

Your Notes

Anny's Teaching

The Container Technique

Ask your client to imagine a container at their left-hand side (I am sitting at my client's right-hand side) and remove all the residues, physical and emotional scars as a result of the issue they just reviewed and put it in the container.

Ask the client, "Anything else you wish to put in the container?" Have the client put a lid on the container and close it tight.

Ask the client what they want to do with what is in the container: transform it into something positive for them now, or dispose of it.

Since there was a lot of energy invested in what is now in the container, I prefer that they want to transform what is in the container into something else.

Transformation

Have the client write the instructions *"to be transformed into"* on the side of the container and send the container to the sun, "to be consumed and transformed into the new energy (or attitude, or feeling, depending on the client's requests), and once it has been transformed, you will have a new, delightful feeling, and when you have it, let me know ..."

Watch your client carefully and be prepared to collapse all the anchors you have established during the session. As the new feeling is coming to them, the breathing changes, and then you say "this new feeling, how does it feel?" Repeat the client and add, breathe it in, breathe it in, and impregnate every cell of your body with the (repeat client) feeling. BREATHE IT IN. As the client breathes the feeling IN collapse the anchors, at the end, letting go as they breathe in the good feeling.

Your Notes

Anny's Teaching

At the end of this exercise, I am deepening the client's trance to go very deep into relaxation, repeating the suggestions.

At that point, I am wrapping up the session repeating the client's description of the good feeling again. There is a page called "Anny's vernacular" so you can use it if you feel it is appropriate. The whole exercise flows well and takes anything from 15 to 30 minutes, depending on the type of session the client has experienced.

Your Notes

Anny's Teaching

Dispose Of The Box And What It Contains

If they want to dispose of "it" instead of sending it to the sun to be burned, consumed and transformed, I sometimes ask them how they want to do it.

Method – 1 – Helium Balloons

If there is an Inner Child or several Inner Children involved, I ask the client to gather a lot of helium balloons so they can lift the box... After all, this is a celebration!

Securely attach the box as close as possible to the balloons and notice the exceptionally long string hanging from the box.

Split the number of strings between the Inner Child / Children and Client and start to give the balloons "some strings" and watch it as the balloons are lifting the box with all that stuff inside.

As they all watch the balloons taking the box away for good, I ask client to observe who is letting go first of the strings attached to the box with all that stuff, and who is the last one to let it go is. The verbal feedback on that observation will be revealing to you!

As they are watching the balloons taking the box away for good, I ask client to watch as the balloons are higher and higher and further and further away and wave it goodbye, knowing that by the time they are back home (or anything within a time frame) the box will be gone for good.

At the end of this exercise, I am deepening the client's trance to go very deep into relaxation, repeating the suggestions.

Your Notes

Anny's Teaching

At that point, I am wrapping up the session repeating the client again. Ass you know, there is a page called "Anny's vernacular" so you can use it if you feel it is appropriate. The whole exercise flows well and takes anything from 15 to 30 minutes, depending on the type of session the client has experienced.

Method – 2 – Hot Air Balloon

Ask the client to put the box in the basket, the gondola, of a hot air balloon, then step back and watch as the burner of the hot air balloon is fired up, hear the burner filling up the balloon with hot air. As the client and anyone else involved in the healing are watching, the balloon is getting fuller and fuller of hot air, straightening itself up and starts to pull on the ropes attached to the gondola with the box in it.

As they are watching the balloon taking the box away for good, I ask client to watch as the balloon is higher and higher and further and further away and wave it goodbye, knowing that by the time they are back home (or anything within a time frame) the box will be gone for good.

At the end of this exercise, I am deepening the client's trance to go very deep into relaxation, repeating the suggestions.

At that point, I am wrapping up the session repeating the client again. As you know, there is a page called "Anny's vernacular" so you can use it if you feel it is appropriate. The whole exercise flows well and takes anything from 15 to 30 minutes, depending on the type of session the client has experienced.

There are sometimes other methods requested by clients.

Your Notes

Anny's Teaching

What To Do When A Client Gets Into Distress

Sometimes, a client in great distress comes for a session, sobbing.

What I do then is doing an emotional stress release. This usually turns into a complete session since I do it until the client calms down and then can view and clearly understand the situation that was upsetting them.

For your sake, please remember to "download" through your feet the energy the client is releasing.

As I explained to you before, over the years, I had to remove myself twice for about 30 second, the energy so intense I almost passed out.
It was twice about an accident with a horse.

During a session, a client sometimes becomes agitated emotionally, mixings situations, events and losing clarity of thoughts.

When that happens, I put my hand gently on their forehead. Slowly moving their head left and right, I say 'let your mind go clear' as I make them breathe though what was triggered.

When stopping breathing you know the client resists releasing what was triggered and is holding on to whatever was triggered.

After having breath through what was triggered and experiencing a profound relieve, the result is feeling much, much better when contemplating what was triggered.

Your Notes

Anny's Teaching

Emotionality Scale

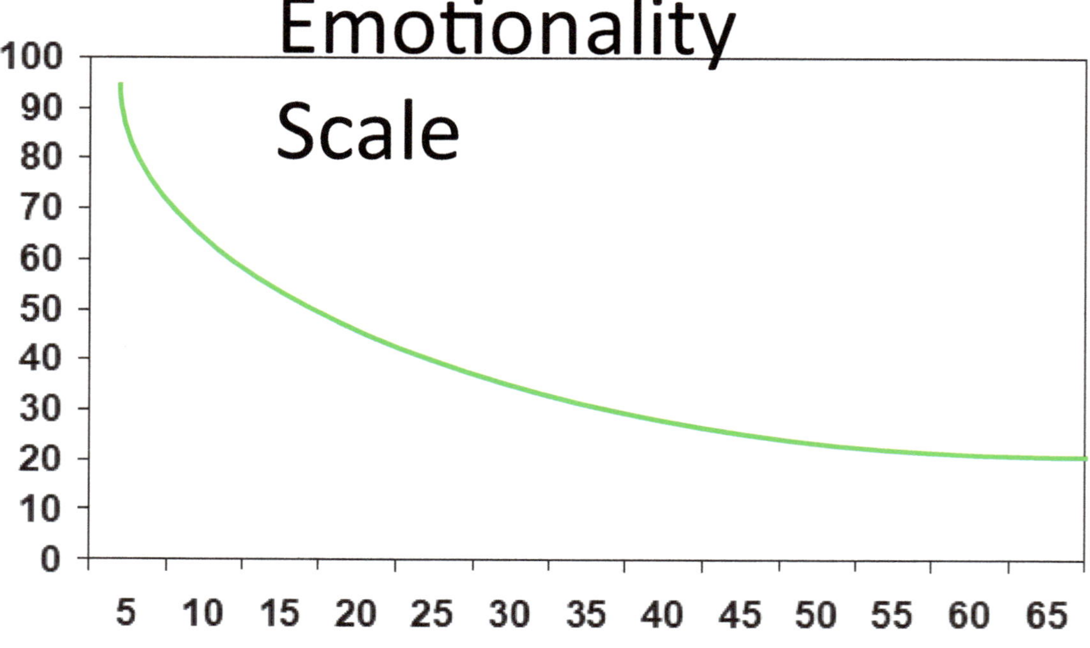

Your Notes

Anny's Teaching

Family Dynamics And How To Navigate The Emotionality Scale

The following is a recreation of the actual session notes that I took along with my annotations. The client's name and a few other items have been changed or omitted to preserve privacy.

You will notice how a child is the catalyst to bring up often painful memories hidden at subconscious level.

Client's name

Date: December 2, 2017

OUT: 11:20
IN: 10:10 am
Time: 1 hour 10

Clients Date of Birth
Client is 52

Reason for session:

- Feels uncomfortable with himself
- Anxious and depressed

May 2016 51 Suicidal. Hospitalised for 3 weeks

20 Married. She was 19

3 daughters: 30 – 29 – 27
(please note how the client started with the oldest daughter)

23 She left

35 Common-law. She was 38

2 stepsons 30 – 28
(please note how the client started again with the oldest stepson)

29? Here I asked what happened when he (the client) was 29.

Questions About John's Session

- Question 1 -
- Question 2 -
- Question 3 -
- Question 4 -
- Question 5 -

Transcript – John's Session – Self Confidence

Anny's Notes:

Client is 14

Out 2:30 pm

In 1:00 pm

Total Time 1:30 hrs

Low self-confidence & self esteem
Trouble sleeping
Lots of time starts and then backs of.

John was **14** at the time of this session.

Interviewing The Mother

His mother had a lot of concern because John was showing the same tendencies as her brother who had committed suicide at age 30: low self-confidence and self-esteem, trouble sleeping and standing back lots of times.

Although things at school were going well, John seemed to start something, knowing he could do it, and then stopped and stood back.

As the interview was going on, I could sense a going forward motion, a fear, then a standing back. So, I asked the mother, "Tell me about his birth."

The delightful mother then became very agitated and explained to me she truly wanted the child. Prior to his birth she had several miscarriages and did everything possible to carry John to term. When she finished, I asked again, "Tell me about his birth." She explained then that John had the umbilical cord wrapped around his neck two times and had to come out by forceps and was not given to his mother for 20 to 30 minutes.

Then I interviewed John

John explained that he likes basketball a lot. It is fun. He plays it since age seven or eight. The coach kept telling John to trust his ability to play well. John kept questioning this, especially when other players were taller than he was.

When asked, "What do you want me to help you with?" John replied without hesitation, **"More self-esteem so I know I can do it."**

Always adjust the induction to the client. Teenagers are usually not trusting and will not co-operate if you ask then to close their eyes. In this case, having asked the permission to touch his knees, eyes wide open, John was very gently lead into a trance by making him talk about the way he felt as he was talking to me, all by himself, sitting in the chair, wired up for sound.

The session had already started as I clicked on 'recording'.

Transcript of John's Session

Anny: Go straight into the feeling.
That feeling there.

I am not sure what you are going to do.
So go inside, just go inside. Go inside the feeling. Go inside the feeling.

And talk to it the way you would talk to a person. After all, it is a part of you, is it not? Explain to it that you understand the feeling. You understand it.

And now ask the feeling "When you feel that way, how old are you in the feeling?"
Go inside and ask the feeling. "When you feel that way, how old are you in that feeling?" Just go in it.
Just go in it. And something is going to come to you. And tell me what comes to you.

When you feel that way, how old do you feel inside?
You are not sure what I am going to do to you.

John: Scared.

Anny: Right. Go into the scared feeling. How old is John that feels scared like that? Go inside the feeling.

It is going to be very interesting. Very interesting.

How old is John?

John: Fourteen.

Anny: Okay, very good. Never felt that way before.

John: Scared? Yah I felt scared before.

Anny: Okay. Go back into the times when you felt scared like that before. Just go in there and just tell me what comes to you.

And trust the information.

John: When I got lost.

Anny: You got lost. How old were you?

John: Ahhh, about five.

Anny: You were five and you got lost. You felt scared like that.

Can you see yourself at five, or can you pretend you see yourself at five?

John: I cannot see myself at five.

Anny: You can pretend?

John: Yah, I remember.

Anny: You remember.

All right.

In your imagination, take the five year old John in your arms, and give him a hug.

Now, as you are taking slow deep breaths, that feeling, that scared feeling, let it come to you quite strongly. And have you ever felt scared like that before? Have you ever felt scared like that before?

John: Yes.

Anny: Ummm humm. And when you feel scared like that, stay with the five-year-old who got scared.

John: Got lost.

Anny: Got lost. Right.

Where were you lost at five?

John: At the store.

Anny: At the store. What type of a store?

John: A grocery store.

Anny: A grocery store.

Five years old, that is pretty scary. Umm humm.
And what happened after that?

John: Ahhh. I kept on walking. Walking up and down the rows.

Anny: Ummm humm. And?

John: And I could not find them.

Anny: And?

John: And then they found me.

Anny: They found you.

How did it feel when they found you?

John: I was relieved.

Anny: Mmmm hummm. Do you remember how that felt, the relief?

John: Yes.

Anny: All right. What a relief huh.

You talk about "them", who were they?

John: My parents.

Anny: Umm humm. Very good.

So make sure the little five-year-old inside of you knows how it ended.
Ummm humm.

And then open your eyes.

How did that feel?

John: When I was lost?

Anny: No, no, the whole exercise?

John: Ahhh.

Anny: How did that feel, to be able to go back as a five year old lost in a store?

John: Quite a difference.

Anny: Ummm humm.

That is what we do here, okay.
There is always a beginning to everything.

And that is what I do here. You got, got the idea now? How does it feel now that you got that idea?

John: Uhhh, kinda relieved.

Anny: Ummm humm. That is what I do here.

For example, you told me, you want to **know you can do it**.

That feeling, John; you know, you want more **self-esteem** so you **know you can do it**.

The fact that you do not **know you can do it** comes from somewhere, so that we can rearrange the memory, so that you know that it was then, and now, John is 14.

For example, take a deep breath, and as you exhale, go back to the little boy, lost in the grocery store, and pretend you see him.

So, take him in your arms, and explain to him how it ended. What a relief right. Now, explain to him that you are 14 now. And that now you go to the store all by yourself.

Updating Inner Child:

Take the five year old little boy in your arms, and show him how things are different from your point of view now, because you are much stronger.

Right? It makes a difference, huh?
Now for you to understand how the little boy felt at five, when he, you know in that store, just crouch down, so that you can see things from his eye level.

And look at the shelves. Look at the people. Look at those baskets in the grocery store. Look at that.

Can you see the difference?

John: Yes.

Anny: Okay. So, you get to stand up again, and take the little boy in your arms, so that he knows how tall you are now. And make sure he knows that you can go shopping all by yourself.

And if you have the memory of something you bought all by yourself and it was a lot of fun to buy in a store … in your imagination, take the little five-year-old John with you, and go into that store.

And show him the fun you had in buying something that was very special to you. And then give the little boy a hug and explain to him that is the pleasure of being a grown-up.

And then open your eyes.
Alright. How was that?

John: Better than the first time.

Anny: Ummmm hummm.

That is because the scare was still the scare of a five-year-old.

Now you brought it up to date. Now you are 14.

Can you tell the difference? By the way, can you share with me what you went to the store for to buy, that was lots of fun to buy?

John: Candy.

Anny: Candy.

Very good. Ummm humm. Yah. And you can do it all by yourself, do you?

John: Yup.

Anny: And you know how to count and get the change, make sure you got the correct change, right?

John: Yup.

Anny: Umm humm.

That is what I do here all the time. So now, I would like you to think about when you are five-year-old, lost in that store.

Checking my work:

Now that you think about it, how does it feel?

John: Kind of silly that you can get lost.

Anny: Right.

John: At the store.

Anny: Mind you, you understand the five-year-old, do you?

John: Yah.

Anny: Okay, this is what I do here, I make you understand things and leave the memory intact, because that is part of you.

To have been lost at five in the store is part of you, right?

However, now, at 14, you look back and it feels different, because you are 14 now.

Going after the issue:

So … I wonder what happened with your **self-esteem**.
What is it that at one point you wanted to do, and you got scared because you **could not make it**.

What is it?

As I am saying that, I would like you to feel your body. Just be very sensitive of your body. Your body feelings there.

And as I am saying that, you are going to have the part of your body who is going to become more – how can I explain that – that you will become more aware of, as I am saying that. There is one time that very scared you thought you **would not make it.**

There was one time.

There is part of your body is going to be more… you are going to become more aware of a part of your body as I saying it.

There is one time when you thought you **would not make it**.

Ummm humm. You thought, my God, **I will not make it.**

I will not make it. I will not make it. What part of your body is starting to really become more sensitive?

You will not make it.

John: My arms.

Anny: Ummm humm, your arms. Go into your arms. Go into the feeling in your arms. Go into that feeling. Just sink into it and thank the feeling for coming to you.

Thank the feelings for coming to you.

And stay with the feelings, John, stay with the feelings, stay with the feelings and go inside the feeling and ask the feeling "Where were you when it felt that way? and trust what comes to you.

Go into the feeling, the feeling will give you that information. And even if it does not make sense to you, tell me what comes.

What is going on that your arms feel like that?

John: I am caught in a rope.

Anny: You are caught in a rope. You are caught in a rope. All right, repeat that. I am caught in a rope.

John: I am caught in a rope.

Anny: You are caught in a rope.

John: I am caught in a rope.

Anny: Where are you, subconscious mind? Where is he?

Where is he?

He is caught in a rope, where is he? Come on.

The first thing. Trust it. Trust it.

John: It is up high.

Anny: It is up high. You are right. And?

John: Stuck.

Anny: Stuck, right.

Thank the feeling. Thank the feeling.

So you are caught in a rope, high, up high, you are stuck.
Any other feelings?

Any other feelings?

You are stuck. You are stuck. And what is coming to mind as you feel that way?

You are stuck. You are stuck.

John: I am never going to get down.

Anny: You are never going to get down.

Never going to get down. Right.

Where are you?

Where are you? Just trust what comes.

Look around you. Look around you.

Look around you and trust what comes.

Of the feelings on your body. Of the feelings on your body.

Tell me where you are.

John: Outside.

Anny: You are outside, okay. And?

John: There is a rope there.

Anny: Ummm humm.

In your imagination, look down at your feet.

Where are you?

John: High up.

Anny: High up. Right. High up.

What time of the year is it?

Feel the sense, the temperature on your body.

John: Summer.

Anny: Summer. All right.

You are going to feel the feelings on your body.

It is summer. Day or night?

John: Day.

Anny: It is what?

John: Day.

Anny: It is day.

Are you alone or with someone?
First thing (snap fingers). First thing.

John: I am alone.

Anny: You are alone.

Okay, You are going to rewind the movie of time.

How did you get there?

Rewind the movie of time a little bit. How did you get there?

First thing that comes to you.

John: I was walking.

Anny: You are walking.

How come you got in the rope, high up?

John: I tried to climb it.

Anny: You tried to climb it.

How old are you?

First thing that comes.

John: Seven.

Anny: You are seven.

And the rope, huh.
Where is the rope caught?

John: In a tree.

Anny: And on your body, where is it?

John: It is around my arms.

Anny: Around your arms.

How come it caught around your arms?

Rewind the movie of time so that you will know how you got in that situation.

John: I started wiggling.

Anny: You started wiggling. And?

John: Got caught. It got wrapped around my arms.

Anny: Ummm humm. Very good.

As you take a deep breath and exhale, "My God**, I will not make it"**, I will never come down!"

Subconscious mind, subconscious mind, same feeling, another time.

Same feeling, subconscious mind, another time.

"My God, I will not get down. I will not get down".

"I am caught. I am caught. I will not get down. I will not get down."

First thing that comes to you, John. Even if it does not make any sense tell me.

John: What?

Anny: Another situation when you felt the same way.

So stay with the feelings and the feelings will bring you right back to another time when you felt that way, even if it does not make sense to you John.

Trust the feelings. The information is in the feeling.

Feeling caught like that. The rope is around you. You will never get down. Feeling caught like that. "My God, **I will not make it!**"

Talk.

John: I cannot think of anything.

Anny: That is because you think. A feeling does not think John.

So come back to the seven-year-old caught in the rope.

Climbed the tree, right?

And you got caught, humm? In the rope? Started to wiggle humm.

Pretend you enter into the picture now, and you help the seven year old John.

Help him.

Be kind to him and have good humour. Very good humour. Be kind to this little boy.

So help him untangle himself, right, and make sure he is safe.

And by the way, John, how did that event end up? When you got caught there in a tree. How did you untangle yourself?

John: Well, I just stopped wiggling and the rope unwound, and I dropped down.

Anny: So you got down all by yourself, did you not? Make sure the little boy knows about that.

Right. Make sure you tell him that, hey, here is the way it was. You did it all by yourself, did you not?.

And explain to him it was just like at five, in the store, getting lost. It ended up right, did it not?

What a relief, huh. Umm humm. What a relief.

Now let us go back to the seven year old who got tangled up in a rope. And make sure you explain to the little boy how the whole thing ended up. When you got to the ground, all by yourself, what happened then?

John: I ran back.

Anny: Where?

John: To where we were staying.

Anny: Alright. And what happened when you got back?

John: Nothing.

Anny: Did you tell you mom and dad? Were your mom and dad there, or were you with other people?

John: My Dad was there.

Anny: Your Dad was there. So did you tell him?

John: Yah, I just told him that I kind of got caught in a tree there and I got down.

Anny: And what did he say?

John: He asked me how I got caught and all that.

Anny: Umm humm.

John: And he asked me if I was hurt or anything.

Anny: Ummm humm. And?

John: No.

Anny: Alright. Very good.

Make sure the seven-year-old knows that everything was all right. And guess what? You did it yourself.

And then open your eyes. How was that?

John: It felt different than the two times before.

Anny: How different?

John: Uhhh, it was a little scarier.

Anny: Umm humm. And when the ending was good, how was it?

John: Ahhh, it was a relief that I got down.

Anny: Umm humm. Did you know that you could remember so well, hey? Humm.

All right. Take a slow deep breath, and as you exhale, realize that although the second time was scarier than the third time was scarier than the first two times, you did very well did you not? And the ending was good. Ummm humm.

So, take a slow deep breath and as you exhale, get the feeling again. Get that feeling again "My God, **I will never make it**," you know, that scary feeling.

That scary feeling. That scary feeling. Let it come again.
Let it come again. That is right.

And you are going, again, to become very, very much aware of feelings on your body.

"My God, **I will never make it**. My God **I will never make it**."

Let it come to you. Let it come to you.

"Oh my God, **I will never make it. I will never make it."**

And become aware of your body. And you are going to have a sensation in your body and you are going. Where is it?

And trust the information. Always trust your feelings John.

John: In my feet.

Anny: Your feet.

All right. Take a slow deep breath and as you exhale, go into the feeling in your feet. And thank it for coming.

"My God, **I will never make it**."

Your feet. Your feet.

Now, as you take a slow deep breath and exhale, just sink into the feeling in your feet.

Sink into the feeling.

Sink into it and ask your feet "What's going on that it feels that way?

"My God, **you will never make it**."
Your feet. What is going on? What is going on?

John: They hurt.

Anny: They hurt. All right. They hurt.

John: They hurt.

Anny: They hurt. All right, they hurt.

John: Hurt.

Anny: They hurt. What did they hear? Very good. They hurt. What did they hear?

Go inside, go inside and trust yourself. What is it here? Trust the feeling.

John: Running.

Anny: Huh?

John: I was running.

Anny: You were running.

And what is going on, you are running? What is going on?

"My God, **you will never make it**".

"My God, **you will never make it!"**

John: Something is behind me.

Anny: Something is behind you.

Get the feel of where you are. Where you are, something is behind you.

How old are you? First thing. (snap fingers)

John: Nine.

Anny: You are nine. Okay. And what is going on?

John: A dog is chasing me.

Anny: A dog is chasing you.

A dog is chasing you. Is it night or day?

John: It is day.

Anny: It is day. Morning or afternoon?

John: Afternoon.

Anny: Umm humm.

"My God, **you will never make it!** My God, **you will never make it!"**

Now, run next to the little boy Well he is not that little any more. And he is running.

Run beside him and go to the end of the story. Tell me what happened.

John: The person who owned the dog, whistles and called it back and it ran back to him. And I ran into the house, our house.

Anny: How did it feel when the dog got called and it ran back? How did it feel?

John: I felt really happy when it was gone to its owners.

Anny: Right. Now, and then you got to the house. Who was there?

John: My Mom.

Anny: Did you tell her? And what did she say?

John: Well, when I came running into the house screaming and she asked what was wrong. And I told her about the dog.

Anny: Yahhh. You were screaming, huh.

You were screaming. You were screaming.

Now, turn around and take the nine-year-old boy with you now. Ask him to look at you. You are 14 now. You are 14 now.

Umm humm. And point out how it ended up. You were safe, did you not?

Umm humm. Make sure he knows, the nine-year-old knows. And now, John, when you are playing basketball, get … , it is a court of what, how do you call that?

John: Court.

Anny: Go to the court with your team and ask the four year old, the five year old, the seven year old, and the nine year old John to sit there and watch you.

And explain to them it is like all the other memories. **You made it.**

And when you play basketball you play for the fun of it. And it does not matter how tall or short a person is, **you will make it.** Because you know from all the experience you had before that **you did make it**, did you not?. Explain that.

Imagine they are all four there and explain it to them. **You made it**, did you not? Explain it to them.
So now, when you go on the court there, you step on the court or anywhere else, when you know you want something, trust yourself.
Remember that each time you got in a situation **you made it,** did you not?.
Remember the first time you got scared, **you made it**.

Remember being lost in the store - **you made it.**

Hummm. Caught in a tree – well **you made it all right**.

Even the dog? You were a pretty good runner, did you not? Right.

Make sure they, all four, they know that from now on when you go on the court, you step on the court or any other situation when **self-esteem** is required, that you remember that every time **you made it**. Thank you very much.

And when you are finished, open your eyes. Just give them a good lecture, and put some fun in there. Laughter is very good medicine. So just let them realize that.

How was that?

John: Good. It was … fine. That was just as good as the previous one.

Anny: You are right. How different was it, according to you?

John: Umm … different because, ahhh, nothing really bad happened.

Anny: It all went, ended up fine, did it not?

John: Yup.

Anny: Right. And now when you look back, some are really funny, do you not think so?

Ahh, it was not funny at the time, not at all. You know.

But when you look back, you say "Come on", huh.
So from now on, remember that **you made it** every time, because you got it - you have the make-up for it.
Do you understand what I am saying?

Now. Would you like to experience hypnosis?

John: Sure.

Anny: Alright. Trust me enough for that?

John: Yah.

Anny: It is going to be simply for relaxation.

Note:
Remembering his mother concerns about John's trouble sleeping.

And tonight, and every night that you, when you are in bed, ready to fall asleep, with your head on your pillow, all what you will have to do is remember that you were here - pretend you are in this office, in this chair, listening to my voice and following instructions.

That is all what you have to do. Then you will take a deep breath, and as you exhale you will close your eyes, and you will go in a wonderful slumber, and you will wake up the next day on time, feeling refreshed, relaxed, renewed, at peace with yourself and with the world around you.

Is that alright with you?

John: Yah.

Anny: Alright.
Well, John, I would like you to look here, keep your eyes here (pointing on the bridge of my nose) and take deep breaths.

I am going to count from one to five and at five your eyelids will be shut tight. Okay.

One, eyelids heavy, droopy.
Two, each time you blink it is hypnosis coming upon you.

Three, your eyelids are getting so heavy, so droopy.

That is right. Four, you can feel it.

So, five, close your eyes, and let all your cares fade away, fade away, fade away.

Let all your cares fade away, fade away, fade away.

And now, I am asking for your protection and your wellbeing, and I say "God, please allow good things to come to John.".

And for this blessing we give thanks."

And now, you ask to be placed into the protection of the light, and, as it is so, inside of you there is a light.

It is the spark of life that is within you.

That spark of life is what makes you breathe, what makes your heart beat, all kind of things like that. What makes you able to feel comfortable or uncomfortable. What makes you feel happy or unhappy. There is an energy inside of you and it is like a light. And let it shine, let it shine. Let it shine throughout every cell of your body, throughout your aura, that energy field around you, strengthening your body, strengthening your aura, strengthening your **self-esteem**, and mentally repeat with me: "This is my body. This is my space. Only light can come from me. Only light can come to me. Only my light can be here".

And now …

You are on the tenth floor and you are going to go down to the first floor and when you reach the first floor you will find something, even if you are not aware of it now, it will be there for you. It is something about you that will give you **self-esteem**, self-confidence.

I should rephrase that.

As the door will open on the first floor, you will find there something about you. It is something about you. And by finding it again, because you had it before, it will give you a lot of **self-esteem** and self-confidence, inner peace, and inner joy. It is a part of you that you are going to find again. And even if you are not aware of it, it will be there, and it will come to you. Even if you are not aware of it.

So now, here you are on the tenth floor, in front of an elevator. You punch the button so that you call the elevator.

Then, here is the elevator and the door opens, and wow, this is the perfect elevator. You never thought it was possible to have an elevator like that. You like the walls of the elevator. It is exactly what you like. It is the music that relaxes you.

So you step into the elevator. You notice that you are on the tenth floor and you want to go to the first floor, so you punch one. The door closes and there is something to sit on it or lay down on it. Whatever it is. Something you really like.

So, you get on it, and you are enjoying the ride, listening to the music.

And as you are going down, down, deeper and deeper, and as the floors are passing, one after the other, you are going down, down, you become so relaxed, so relaxed.

You are enjoying every minute of it. Every minute of it. You really are enjoying it.

And now you can tell you are going to reach floor number one.

And, as the elevator stops, you feel so relaxed that you do not feel like coming out of it.

The doors open, and here it is. Whatever it is, it is a part of you here that you did not know you had.
It is giving you back your **self-esteem**, your self-love, inner peace, great joy, and I am asking your subconscious mind, open and receptive to the suggestions you are receiving now, to sort all things out, and reveal to you what it feels you should know and understand.

And I am asking your subconscious mind to reveal it to you in a way that you will remember and understand. And the information will come to you at the most unexpected times, much to your surprise and delight.

Much to your surprise and delight.

You are more relaxed that you have been for a while, and each time you enter this type of relaxation you will enjoy a deeper and better quality of relaxation, giving you a lot of joy, peace of mind, self-confidence, **self-esteem**, inner peace again. Feeling great, feeling great to be alive.

And I am asking your subconscious mind, open and receptive to the suggestions you are receiving now, to make all the necessary changes now, so that all this or something even better now manifests itself in your attitude, your behavior, your life, in a most successful, satisfying, gracious, diplomatic, and joyful way.

And the benefits of this session and all the counselling you had prior to this session will stay with you for hours, days, weeks, months, and years to come, much to your surprise and delight.

And when you are ready John, you will take a very deep breath, open your eyes, and stretch.

And tonight, and every night, when you are in bed with your head on your pillow, ready to fall asleep, all what you will have to do is remember being here, feeling so great, so relaxed, in many ways.

And as you are remembering listening to my voice, all what you will have to do is take a slow deep breath and as you exhale, you will close your eyes and remember how relaxed you were in this office and you will enjoy a wonderful slumber, to wake up on time, feeling refreshed, relaxed, renewed, feeling great in every way.

And when you are ready, you will take a deep breath now, fill up your lungs, open your eyes, and stretch.

How was that John?

John: Fine.

Anny: Did you enjoy it?

John: Yup.

Anny: Now. You remember everything, do you not? Anything you want to share with me. Up to you.

John: Ummm. No.

Anny: Did you surprise yourself, John?

John: Umm. Sort of, I guess.

Anny: Can you share with me how you surprised yourself?

John: Umm. Well, I really did not know like why.

Like I knew those things happened, but I did not really like remember them that well.

Like right now, I still do not like dogs. Like big ones. I just never really knew why and all that.

Anny: Okay.

John: Uhhh, stuff like that.

Anny: Are you making more sense to yourself now?

John: Yah.

Anny: Umm humm. Feels better, huh? Yah. That is all for today then. Okay.

Questions About Nathan's First Session

- Question 1 -

- Question 2 -

- Question 3 -

- Question 4 -

- Question 5 -

Transcript – Nathan's First Session – Skin Rash

OUT 5:50pm Client will be 15 next month

IN 4:20pm

Wore the same 2 shirts since Grade 6

1h ½ Started at **11**

The Interview with the father

I first talked to the client's father to know what is his concern.

Client is wearing the same 2 shirts since Grade 6.

Client complains wearing a shirt irritates his skin – chest and neck and upper arms – and it hurts.

Client's father complained that, when playing football, Nathan wears the team's uniform and feels fine. A shirt is something else, and when he wears a good one, insist at putting one of his ragged shirts under it, and pulls the ragged collar up over the good shirt to protect his neck, for everyone to see. This is most embarrassing to both parents.

Client's father explained they went all over in an attempt to fix the shirt-hurt problem: Family physician, skin specialist, psychologist and even psychiatrist, with no results. So decided to bring Nathan to me for hypnosis sessions.

When Nathan came to my office escorted by his father, he was wearing a T-shirt, clean and falling apart, with holes all over, it so worn out.

The Interview with Nathan

Once alone with Nathan, I asked him to give me his side of the story.

He promptly explained that when he puts on a shirt, everywhere it touches, it hurts. Usually on the torso. It is like a burning sensation.

He likes something that has been worn for a while.

Client explained it started in Grade 1, when his mother told him "You are going to wear that shirt".

Bothered when "FORCED" to wear the shirt.

The rest of my notes can be read in the transcript of the session.

Transcript of Nathan's first session

Anny: Now Nathan, I am going to explain to you what I do here.

As I am talking and so forth and you are talking, especially when you are talking, I am using a technique that is called anchoring. It is a technique that is used in many ways and the way I use it, I will be touching your knees and it will be firm touch like that.

Sometimes I will touch this knee. Sometimes the other. Sometimes both.

And I would like your permission to do so.

Nathan: Okay, go ahead.

Anny: Well, yes, they are your knees you know, and I am quite respectful of my clients. So, I want permission. Okay, well thank you for that. Just put your head back. That is okay.

So, while I am going to do that so that it is easier on your eyes. (Dimming the light.)

What happened? When were you wearing that shirt the first time?

Nathan Umh, it was at a day camp a few years ago.

Anny: Okay first time, one of the first time.

Nathan: Yes, because it was actually the first time my Mom brought it for me.

Anny: Ohh. First time you wore what you can call a tee shirt at a day camp.
Tell me about that day camp.

Nathan: Umh, well there was a lot of kids and we had gone to the pool pretty much every day. And yah, we were supposed to be golfing too. It was supposed to be something that we can do during the summer because my Mom worked night shifts, so she slept during the day.

Anny: Okay. All right. Tell me about that day camp. Did you like it? Did you not like it? Whatever.

Nathan: Well, it was okay. I did not really like the teachers that much, but I liked to do the activities.

Anny: Liked the activities? You did not like the teacher too much - huh?

Nathan: They treated us too much like little kids.

Anny: Well at 12 years old, we are not kids any more. Um hum.

Okay, tell me more about that day camp because obviously there is something about the day camp and the shirt, so I would like to know a little more. Tell me.

Nathan: Umh, well I really do not much to tell. I cannot really remember that much about it. It was in this place where I used to play hockey. It was called the Sherwood Park Arena or something like that and there was just a little gym where we would stay for about the whole day until we went off to the pool or to the golfing range.

Anny: That is when you wore that shirt for the first time.

Nathan: Yah, she brought it to me. I cannot remember the exact date, but she forced me to wear it pretty much every day.

Anny: She did?

Nathan: And after awhile it started to become comfortable. I did not like it at first.

Anny: You did not like it at first hey?

Nathan: Yeah, maybe that is just because I do not like any shirts of her's, pretty much. Except for a few that I like I got once in a while.

Anny: There was no sleeves on it? Or you cut it?

Nathan: No, there was no sleeves on it.

Anny: Mother made you wear it, but the shirts are hot. Every day huh?

Nathan: Umh, yah, pretty much every day because she said it would be cool when I am out there. Not like cool as in cool cool.

Anny: Yes, I know cool, fresh. It would be nice to wear. Not looking cool. Be cool. Okay.

Nathan: Right.

Anny: All right very good. And the other one? I understand you have two.

Nathan: I actually have about four.

Anny: About four.

Nathan: Yah, there is this other one that does not look anything like this. It is white. The sleeves come down to here and when I first got it, it was in relatively good shape. It had been worn for awhile by a friend of mine actually and he gave it to us. But now it has got tears in the shoulders and holes all through it. Even worse than this one. So, yah.

Anny: How do you feel about that friend who gave you that.

Nathan: Oh, well we were pretty good friends for awhile, but we kinda drifted apart when we started Junior High.

Anny: Well yah okay. Now given by a friend a worn out already?

Nathan: It was not like holly, but it had been worn.

Anny: White, worn out.

Nathan: It has animals on the front of it. Just like a collage of animals. I guess that would not make a difference, but just a description of the shirt.

Anny: All right, tell me about the other one.

Nathan: Umh, there is this one that has sleeves that come down to here. Black sleeves and it has kind of a grey and blue emblem in the front of it. It really does not have any holes, but it is a touch too small for me.

Anny: Ohh, too small. Okay, the third is getting too small huh?

Nathan: Yup.

Anny: With black sleeves, huh?

Nathan: Yup.

Anny: Okay, and the fourth one?

Nathan: Yup, this one has the same kind of sleeves as the other one, except they are blue and it has a white front with a red emblem in the front. It has __________________ , but is not too small for me or anything like that, so. I really do not wear that one very much, but it does not hurt me or anything.

Anny: Now, there is something I would like to know. This one is red. The second one is white. The third one. There is only white, the second one? The one that your friend gave you?

Nathan: Yup, it is pretty much all white.

Anny: And the third one. The one that is getting too small. What are the colors?

Nathan: and grey and a little bit of blue on the front. It was an old one my Dad used to wear too. He gave it to me as a hand-me-down.

Anny: So you would like something that …

Nathan: Has been worn for awhile.

Anny: I would like to know more about this day camp. Do you remember one of the first time you went to day camp?

Nathan: No, not really. I just remember it was either two or even three years ago, maybe when I was 11 even.

Anny: Okay, tell me about it.

Nathan: I am pretty sure I have told all of it. I cannot even really remember the faces or the names of the teachers. I just remember they treated us too much like kids and I did not really like that very much. It kind of reminded me of my first day care when I was six.

Anny: Tell me about that.

Nathan: I did not like that either. There was this woman, Suzy, that was rather mean, I guess.

Anny: She was rather mean. Tell me, how does that feel?

Nathan: Well, I guess that she really was not like really yelling kind of mean, but I just really did not like her how she related to the kids.

Anny: How do you like people to relate to kids?

Nathan: Well, I just do not like them treating them like they are idiots. They do not know what they are talking about or anything like that.

Anny: Well, I will say, I agree. Kids have a mind too. Okay. Because I would like to know what is that is really hurting? What is that is really hurting?

Nathan: Well, what is really hurting with my shirts? I do not know, it just, it feels like a physical pain.

Anny: Oh, I am pretty sure.

Nathan: And it hurts right around in my chest mostly. Right around in here and in the small of my back too.

Anny: Is that right?

Nathan: Yah, when I sit down.

Anny: Yah, I know what you mean.

Nathan: And right where it cuts off at the sleeves. That kind of bothers me. It is not really a pain, but it is kind of a scratchy that is just annoying. I do not know why that would happen, but, yah.

Anny: Okay. Anything else that you feel I should know?

Nathan: I do not really think so. I have had this problem for quite awhile. My Mom thinks that it started in Grade 4, but that is when I think she started to become worried about it. I think I have had it for quite a long time. Pretty much when I started school.

Anny: Ah ha! Had it since starting school. Thank you very much for that information. There is something about it.

Nathan: I remember one time when I was, I think in Grade 1 even. Because I remember my teacher, Mrs. Geffery, being out there and my Mom had brought this shirt. I think I had been bothered by other shirts because I remember saying I do not know why this shirt bothered me before. It was kind of like the sleeves right here were like a turtleneck and it was really bothering me during the day. It had not bothered me at first, but it started to become itchier and itchier and it was hot too during the day. So that really bothered me.

Anny: Okay. You know you are giving me very good information today. Thank you. You are really helping me helping you, let me tell you. Okay you also have a very good memory do you not?

Nathan: Yah, I do, I guess.

Anny: How are things in school?

Nathan: Right now?

Anny: Um hum.

Nathan: Ah, they are pretty good actually. Yah. It is not because I am unpopular because of this or anything. I have quite a few friends and other people just - if they are not my friends, they usually just leave me alone anyway.

Anny: Just like if they are not your friends, you leave them alone too.

Nathan: So, I really do not have any enemies there or anything like that.

Anny: Okay. All right. There are many things that I can - I know what I want to do and there are many ways.

Okay I am going to do it the way I feel in my heart I can do so it is easy on you.

Okay just put your head back. Do you know what I do here?

Nathan: Umm. You hypnotize me.

Anny: Yah, but then only if you want to. And also understand that hypnosis can be used for anything. It is just like this pen. I can write notes here. I can write a love letter. I can write a letter of complaint. I can draw a map how to get here. I can do all kinds of things. It is a tool, and I am using hypnosis as a tool.

Because you see Nathan, whatever it is that really bugs you, you know it. It is inside of you. It is like a journal. We all have a journal and the way I use hypnosis, you will be able to read that journal.

Nathan: Ohhh yah?

Anny: Only you will know what is in that journal because there is something about it. There is really something about it. How would it be if you could wear anything you want and feel comfortable?

Nathan: It actually much better. I would not have any complaints about school actually.

Anny: Would it be great!

Nathan: Yah, that is actually my only complaint about school. I have to wear a shirt if I go there.

Anny: Um hum.

Nathan: Yah, well I mean of course. It bugs me. It is annoying. It kind of hurts my concentration too.

Anny: Okay, that will be good. All right. I am going to ask you... . I am going to be.... Well, I am usually very gentle so, that it is very comfortable for you and remember that everything is recorded so if later you want to check things out, you can. And you will remember anyway. I make sure you do. Oh yah, because otherwise you know, how can you talk to me. Because the only person who has all the information is you, you know. So, I am going to help that information come to you, so that you know what is this all about. So life can be much, much easier on you. Okay? Is that fair enough?

Nathan: Yes, that is really what I want, so yah.

Anny: So, I am going to ask you since you think from what your memory is, it started when you started to go to school?

Nathan: Yah.

Anny: Do you remember which school it was?

Nathan: Westbury Elementary.

Anny: Swell. Okay, very good.

Nathan: Yah, that is pretty much the only school I have been. Yah, the problem started here. When I came to Alberta. Well we moved from Ontario to Alberta and I pretty much started kindergarten. I do not recall any problems, but that was quite a few years ago, really. Maybe I just do not remember.

Anny: So problems start?

Nathan: It started in like Grade 1. Pretty much Grade 1.

Anny: Grade 1. And just moved from Ontario.

Nathan: Yah, just one year out of Ontario, we were in.

Anny: One year out of Ontario. Have you gone to Ontario since?

Nathan: Yep. We have all of our relatives are out there actually.

Anny: Is that right? Okay, where in Ontario, because you know I come from Ontario too and I know where Ontario is.

Nathan: Is quite big

Anny: Where in Ontario?

Nathan: Our grandparents live in Sarnia and my uncle and my cousin and my aunt live out in London.

Anny: Okay, very good. All right. Warmer over there, especially this year, it is quite cold here.

Nathan: Yah.

Anny: But usually over there it is quite nice. So, London, Ontario and Sarnia would be quite nice. Sarnia - where is that again? Just a moment, I used to live in Ontario so I could pick Sarnia here and I am going to refresh my memory. Okay, do you remember - how old were you then?

Nathan: I was about 5, I think. Maybe just turning 6. Because I remember we left shortly after my birthday.

Anny: So that makes it easy to remember. So in June, huh? Do you remember that? Go back there. Just close your eyes and go back there.

Nathan: To Ontario or to my birthday?

Anny: No, no. Well okay, go to your birthday. No, I said close your eyes, but you know what if you do not want to close your eyes, that is fine too. I am quite all right with that. It is simply for some people it is easier, so you decide, is it easier to do it when you have your eyes closed, or is it easier to do it when they are not closed? I would like you to go back to that particular birthday.

Nathan: Well, I do not really remember that much. Um, I remember getting some presents. This little teenage mutant ninja turtle's thing that I used to play with a lot.

Anny: Okay, good. Do you remember who was there?

Nathan: God, I cannot think of his name. I think it was like Peter.

Anny: Is it is a cousin, or is it a friend?

Nathan: It was a close friend who had lived across the street of us.

Anny: Okay, so do you know - when did you know that you were moving to Alberta?

Nathan: I think we had known quite a bit in advance because the plant that my Dad worked at, Dow Chemical, it was closing down there because of all the strikes that had been going on. So we were going to be relocated to the plant in Alberta. So that is why we were moving and I think I knew quite a bit in advance, I am pretty sure.

Anny: Okay and do you remember how it was when you left Ontario? Go back there.

Nathan: I do not remember actually going to the airport, but when I was on the plane, my Dad said I was really quiet the whole time.

Anny: Is that right.

Nathan: Yah, flying out there. I was just looking out the window, I guess.
Anny: So you were very quiet, huh?

Nathan: Maybe I was just sleeping, but I do not know.

Anny: Okay, go back there. Find yourself on the airplane and what is most important, how were you feeling as you were on the airplane flying to Alberta? Go back there.

Nathan: I cannot really quite remember how I felt. I remember looking out the window.

Anny: The feeling is still there. So just trust what comes. Just trust - totally trust.

Nathan: Humm. I think I just did not want to go. I did not want to leave yet.

Anny: You did not want to go. Um hum.

Nathan: I had friends there, so.

Anny: I can hear it through your voice when you talk about it. Yah. Have you seen those friends since?

Nathan: No. I do not think so.

Anny: Okay

Nathan: We were pretty much too young to keep in touch.

Anny: Yah, but it depends. If you go back every year for example, then you do. But if you are going there after five years, well you do not.

Nathan: Yah I know, but yah we did not go back for I think it was like maybe two years after we had left. So I had made friends here, so.

Anny: So go back there. You did not want to go.

Nathan: I was looking out the window. Pretty much the whole time and I think I fell asleep.

Anny: And what was on your mind and what were you thinking and how were you feeling as you looked out the window?

Nathan: Well, it was my first time on a plane too, so.

Anny: Was it?

Nathan: Yah.

Anny: How did you like it?

Nathan: I do not think I was scared or anything like that. It was kind of like just a car or something. I was never afraid of flying or anything like that. But, yah, I am not sure if I was really looking out because I was upset or just that I wanted to see the cars in the clouds.

Anny: Do you remember how you felt as you were on the plane? How did you feel? Go back to it. All the feelings are there. Everything is there.

Nathan: I cannot really dig them up.

Anny: That is all right, that is fine. All right. And now you will advance to the first day of school in Alberta.

Nathan: Okay. The first day of school, I think I was in kindergarten there. And there was this teacher I really liked, Mrs. Wellton.

Anny: You liked her?

Nathan: Yup.

Anny: What was nice about her?

Nathan: She was kind. She was really nice. She did not treat us like we were morons too. She talked to us and read to us, but it was not like she was condescending or anything like that.

Anny: Okay, very good. And then, so here you are. You like that teacher, Mrs. Watson. You have very good memory.

Nathan: Yah, actually yah I guess.

Anny: Yes you do, which is great. And how was teacher in Grade 1.

Nathan: I did not like her. She was quite old actually and she was mean. She yelled too much considering we were in Grade 1.

Anny: She was yelling?

Nathan: Yah, she yelled quite a bit.

Anny: Do you remember how you felt? In your mind, be there as she yells. How does that feel?

Nathan: Well, it was upsetting. She never really yelled at me specifically. I was always a good student, but she would yell a lot at the whole class in general, pretty much.

Anny: And how do you feel when someone yells?

Nathan: I do not really like it that much, but I am usually - I do not know I just - it really does not affect me anymore, I guess.

Anny: Yes, but when you were young?

Nathan: When I was young, yah I guess that would upset me.

Anny: And since the whole thing started when you were young, we are going to go when you were young.

Nathan: Okay, so are - yah.

Anny: Okay. Hum. Do you trust me enough to do some hypnosis.

Nathan: Yah, I guess.

Anny: Is it yes, I guess?

Nathan: Yes, I guess that is why I am here.

Anny: Okay very good. Because I am going to do something. There is something about it because you know I am used to look at people and I can tell that from the time you start to talk about Grade 1 there, something is going on there. Um hum. That was not a pleasant experience.

Nathan: No, I never liked her all through Westborough. She always just seemed kind of mean in my eyes. Probably not a good Grade 1 teacher.

Anny: Wow.

Nathan: Maybe for a later grade.

Anny: But not for Grade 1.

Nathan: More mature.

Anny: Did not have enough patience any more? Okay. Very good. Do you remember how you looked like in Grade 1?

Nathan: Not really actually. I think my hair was actually pretty much the same. Maybe not right now. I had a haircut a couple of days ago. But it was always long and thick. Well not really long, just pretty much thick and I was smaller than I am now.

Anny: Well yeah.

Nathan: Yah, but I mean even for now, I think I got quite a bit bigger because I was pretty small, yah.

Anny: You were pretty small. So, I am going to do something. Remember, just relax. Everything is recorded. Although you remember everything. That thing people do not remember - umh umh. Okay I would like you to, in your mind.... Oh, by the way, do you remember how that school is? How old is that school? Yah, how you got into the school and everything. Do you remember that?

Nathan: Yah, there was a couple of doors on each side. There was about five main doors and then there is the right side, where all the Grade 1 through Grade 4, where we all played. Yah, and we would go through these separate doors to get to our classrooms.

Anny: Where would you leave your coats and everything, especially in the winter?

Nathan: There were little open lockers where we would just hang up our stuff.

Anny: All right. Well, I am going to ask you to do something. In your mind find yourself at home ready to go to school.

Nathan: In Grade 1. Okay humm. There is one time, the time that I had told you about when I had worn that shirt and it was bothering me all through the day. I remember my Mom, she had picked out this shirt and she had said you are going to wear this. Kind of forcefully because I guess I had been fighting with her about wearing shirts before it. I do not really remember all the times of course. I just remember this one time it kind of sticks out in my mind.

Yah. And I put on this shirt and I remember saying that I do not know why this shirt did not bother me before, but when I got to the school it was bugging me all through. Yah, so she had always dressed me and pretty much all the way through, she picks out my clothes and she used to pick out my clothes through elementary.
Now I pretty much just wear the one shirt. This blue shirt with the NAIT logo right here. So yah, she had pretty much picked my shirts out the whole time.

Anny: How do you feel when somebody tells you what to do?

Nathan: It does not really bother me that much. I would have thought that it would have bothered me more. Pretty much the only thing that bothers me about it was that she was forcing me to wear these shirts. It was not really that she was telling me to.

Anny: Forced.

Nathan: Do not get me wrong. My Mom is not a bad person or anything like that.

Anny: Oh, I am not talking about that at all. I know she is a good person. Otherwise and I know that your Father is a good person, otherwise you would not be here.

Nathan: Right.

Anny: It is nothing about what I do. Only good. You know that is the most amazing thing, Nathan, only good people come to see me. Yah.

Nathan: Other people would not take their kids there, right.

Anny: Oh yes, you are the second one today.

Nathan: Oh yah, I mean but mean people who really did not really care about.

Anny: I know your parents are fine. You can tell through. You look pretty well cared for. So okay, in your mind, find yourself ready to go to school in Grade 1. In your mind um hum. And when you got it, simply say, I am there.

Nathan: Okay. Okay, I think I got it. I remember we would put off putting on shirts until the very last minute. After breakfast and we would watch TV a bit too and then like a 10 minutes before we had to go, I would put pretty much everything else on before we had to go with the shirt. We had to contend with the shirt. And then I would put it on and I cannot remember if all of them bothered me or not. Yah.

Anny: Now in your mind, here you are Nathan, almost 15. Who is going to walk little Nathan to school?

Nathan: We were usually driven to school actually.

Anny: Well okay, but you go along with little Nathan.

Nathan: Actually in Grade 1 we had taken the bus. I remember.

Anny: Okay, well you go on the bus. You go along for the ride.

Nathan: I remember that I was usually pretty quiet until my brother came and usually sat next to me. But I was usually pretty quiet while we were going. Especially in Grade 1 because I had not really known that many people there.

Anny: Okay, so in your mind, be on that bus. And you are with Grade 1 Nathan. And you know he is a little boy and he is very small you told me. So now the bus stops at the school and you now hold the hand of little Nathan. No matter what the other people say.
Hold the hand of little Nathan. Because you want to know how he feels. That is how come you hold it in your mind, hold his hand as he gets off the bus. How does he feel?

Nathan: Well, I guess I really was not afraid of school. I mean, I used to go there and I just felt like I had to go there. Because I had to go there I really never felt that I did not want to or anything like that.

Anny: And as you are going into the school, stay with him. Hold his hand, so that you know how he feels. And you are going to become very much - you will notice it very much how little Nathan feels in the classroom when the teacher starts to yell.

Nathan: Well, I just wanted to stay out of it. I felt like.

Anny: That does not tell me how you felt.

Nathan: Yah I know. How did I feel?

Anny: Just go back. How did that feel?

Nathan: I cannot really remember how I felt. I remember I did not like her yelling. She yelled too much. She did it too often. Yah.

Anny: She did it too often, huh? All right.

Nathan: It was like she really did not know that we were Grade 1's that we were not used to school yet, hey.

Anny: Well yah, now it does not matter huh. You are used to school. Nathan, think about everything. Have you ever wondered what happened there. How do you call what is happening with your shirt. Is it an irritation? Is it a pain? What is it? How do you call it?

Nathan: It is a pain.

Anny: It is a pain.

Nathan: And it distracts me from whatever else that I am doing. If I do not have this shirt underneath of it, it is pretty much unbearable and I cannot concentrate on what I am doing.

Anny: So now, I would like you to check your body. What is a pain to you. Check your body and you are going to know where is the pain.

Nathan: Actually I usually have a high tolerance for pain, except for this. It never subsided or anything. I played football, so I am used to it.
Anny: The thing is that what I want to know is just check your body and where is the irritation really. Where does it bug you? Just with your mind, go into your body - where does it bug you?

Nathan: My shirts? Where this pain is?

Anny: I do not know. Just go to your mind and how do you feel. What makes it that really bugs you. There is something about concentration. The whole thing bugs you. It irritates you, which is a pain. Go into your body.

Nathan: Hum. Actually I do not really think is that when I get hit or anything. Not when I get hit-hit. Like when I was in football, it was not really any specific place that hurt more than any other place. But when I am wearing a shirt, it seems like it is right in here. Right in the centre of my chest here.

Anny: Okay go there. Go inside the pain right inside your chest. Just go for it. With your mind, go there. And even put your hand on it, so that the pain knows that you know it is there. Just put it like this. Just be kind to it. It hurts. Um hum. Now, with your mind go into that hurt. Go into that hurt and talk to the pain. To the hurt. Talk to it and ask it what is it that it feels that way. And you know what totally comes to your mind, tell me. It does not matter if it makes sense. If it makes sense, it really does not matter.

Nathan: I am not getting anything.

Anny: Okay, so well let us reinforce it.

Nathan: I know it is there too.

Anny: Stare at my fingers. Listen to my voice. By the way, have you been hypnotized before.

Nathan: No.

Anny: You are going to find that it is extremely pleasant.

Nathan: Okay.

Anny: Really nice. Really pleasant. Stare at my fingers. Listen to my voice. Just keep your gaze on my fingers. Listen to my voice. Your eyelids are getting so heavy. So heavy. Take a slow deep breath and as you exhale, close your eyes and during this experience each time you close your eyes, you relax more and more. More and more.

As I am asking for your protection and your well being and I say God, please allow only good things to come to Nathan, and to me, Anny. And for this blessing, we give thanks,

And now I am going to ask you to put yourself into the protection of a very beautiful light inside of you. At the tip of your heart there is a light. It is like a mini sun in your chest.

Some people can see it. Some people can feel it. Some people simply know that it is there. That light of yours, that very beautiful light of yours, let it shine, let it shine.

Let it shine towards every cell of your body and to help the energy field around you. It is called an aura and I do not know if you know what it is. It is an energy field around you.

And that light of yours, let it shine, let it shine. So that you are within your very own light. Your very own energy field. From the top of your head to the tip of your toes. Feeling really, really great in every way. It is a very beautiful protection and you know that when you are there in that light of yours, you are safe.

And now, as you take a slow breath and exhale with your mind go into that skin thing. Something with that skin thing. With your mind go into it and if that skin thing could talk to you, what would it say? What would it say if that skin thing could talk? Totally trust what comes to your mind, even if it does not make sense to you.

Nathan: It would say shirt hurting.

Anny: Okay. Well, ask the feeling to let you know what is it about the shirt that is hurting.

Nathan: I do not know. It just hurts me.

Anny: Yah, that is okay. Now ask the skin if it remembers feeling hurt like that? Does it remember feeling hurt like that?

Nathan: Every day.

Anny: Every day and how does that feel?

Nathan: It feels very bad. Every day for my entire life since I started school.

Anny: What does that have to do about school? Ask the pain. Ask the pain what does that have to do about school?

Nathan: Every day I go to school I have to wear a shirt.

Anny: And how does it feel that you have to wear a shirt? How does it feel deep, deep, deep down? Deep, deep. deep, deep down - how does it feel to have to wear a shirt?

Nathan: It physically hurts me and I just do not want to wear them. When I am off on weekends or on summer vacation I do not have to wear them. I do not like school because of it.

Anny: Uhm hum. Would you like to like school? It does not matter what type of shirt you are wearing.

Nathan: Yes.

Anny: Would you like that? All right. By the way, do you swim

Nathan: What?

Anny: Do you swim?

Nathan: Do I swim? Not very often.

Anny: Do you know how to swim? Oh, okay.
Well, in your mind, find yourself in a place where you know it is very safe. It could be a cottage and looking at a lake or being near a lake. Getting to swim in a lake and it is at night. A very, very beautiful night.

So you choose - you can be from a cottage, nice and comfortable, looking out at the lake, or at the beach or swimming. You choose and it is a very, very beautiful night. You know some nights there are some nights although it is dark, you can still see where you are, that type of night. Very beautiful. Nice and warm. Very, very nice and warm.

And as you are there, you notice that the sky is beautiful. All the starts in the sky and in your imagination, you pretend that the stars are falling into the water. They touch the water as you are there watching the whole thing and when the stars are touching the water, because the water is like a mirror and you can see the stars in the mirror - in the water - that each time a star touches the water, it makes a crystal sound.

And as you are there watching the whole thing, notice how safe you feel. Notice the temperature on your skin and notice how good you feel as you are watching all that. And you tell yourself that each time a star touches the water, it makes a crystal sound and that with each crystal sound, you become more and more relaxed. More and more relaxed. More and more relaxed. More and more relaxed.

And you like that type of relaxation and you are going to remember how good that feels. And as you are there relaxing so well, you let your body do its perfect work. So as you are relaxing like that, feeling great, going deeper and deeper into relaxation, I am talking to your body now.

Your body knows exactly what the whole thing is all about. Your body knows exactly what was the event and how the event affected you. So now, as you are relaxing, more and more and more with each crystal sound, you are feeling more and more comfortable and I am asking your body to do its perfect work now. To improve whatever has to be improved so that you can wear any shirt you want and feel very, very comfortable.

So that you can wear anything you want and feel very, very comfortable. And for that, I am asking your body to just get rid of whatever emotion, whatever situation, whatever thinking, whatever stress has to be gotten rid of. I am asking your body to really do that. To remove from your system all the impressions so that you can enjoy wearing anything you want and allow yourself to enjoy school.

In your mind just imagine you really feeling comfortable at school, no matter what you wear. And I am asking your body to accept the new decision that you are making now. You told me that it would make a great difference. You would really be able to enjoy school, if you can wear anything and feel comfortable.

And during this experience, the crystal sounds make you more and more and more relaxed. And every muscle, ever nerve, every fibre, every cell is accepting this new decision and it is doing it right now.

So now, as you are here, truly enjoy being relaxed. Truly enjoying the relaxation. In your mind, find yourself going to school now and being totally, totally comfortable. Totally, totally comfortable. So that when you go to High School it is okay too and whatever you want to go after, which would be college or university or a trade school, whatever, you feel great all the time. Being able to concentrate. Being able to concentrate.

So just relax, relax and during this experience the crystal sounds let you go deeper and deeper into relaxation, which is very good for your body, who knows how to do its job. That is right. I am talking to your body now. Your body knows exactly what the whole thing is all about.

What happened and what you started to do. How your body started to respond to the whole situation. I am directing your body to do its perfect work now. I am directing your body to let go of what it needs to let go of. All the old garbage there, the old stuff. All the old ideas. It knows exactly what to let go of and I am directing your body to accept what you are deciding now.

You want to be comfortable at all times with anything you wear. You want to be comfortable at all times with anything you wear and every muscle and every nerve, every fibre, every cell, is accepting this new decision and it is doing it right now.

So just relax, relax, relax, relax. When you relax like that - when you are relaxed like that, it is very good for your body. It is very, very good for your body. So enjoy the relaxation. Enjoy the relaxation and let all your cares fade away, fade away, fade away, fade away, fade away.

And so it is. As your subconscious mind open and very receptive to the suggestions you are receiving now is sorting all things out. And will make all the necessary improvements right now so that you can relax and always feel good in your skin, no matter what you wear. Being able to wear anything, being able to wear anything. And so it is. And so it is.

And enjoy the relaxation and there is something about this type of relaxation: the more you do it, the better the relaxation. That is right. And so it is.

And when you are ready, you will take a slow deep breath, open your eyes and stretch. How was that?

Nathan: That was weird. It was pretty good.

Anny: It was good huh?

Nathan: Yah.

Anny: I said so, and it is true, huh?
Nathan: Um hum.

Anny: It is very pleasant. Now I use it only for relaxation though, but it is very pleasant. Did you like that? Okay I am going to help you get back to now.

Just a moment here. Stare at my fingers. Put your head back. Keep your gaze on my fingers. Take a slow deep breath and as you exhale close your eyes. And now I am going to count from one to five and then I will say your eyes are open Nathan. You are fully aware, feeling refreshed, relaxed, renewed, totally, totally at peace with yourself and with the world around you. Enjoying a sharp mind, a clear head and a tranquil heart

One - slowly, calmly, easy, gently, beginning to return to full awareness once again. Enjoying a sharp mind, a clear head and a tranquil heart.

Two - each muscle in your body is loose, limp, relaxed and you feel wonderfully good. You feel at peace with yourself and with the world around you. Enjoying a sharp mind, a clear head and a tranquil heart.

Four - your eyes begin to feel sparkling clear, as if bathed it is cool spring water.
And now Five - eyelids open. Open your eyes. Take a slow deep breath. Fill up your lungs and give yourself a good stretch.

Does it feel better now? How did it feel to be relaxed like that?

Nathan: It felt weird.

Anny: Tell me about it.

Nathan: It felt like after awhile, it was just my body was kind of not there any more. It felt it was. Yah. It was just really weird.

Anny: Did you like it?

Nathan: Yah.

Anny: It is very pleasant. When it is done the way I do it.

Nathan: Pardon?

Anny: When it is done the way I do it, it is very, very pleasant. As I explained to you before, you can do it in many ways. So.

All right. So now I am going to stop the recording and give it to you.

Questions About Nathan's Second Session

- Question 1 -

- Question 2 -

- Question 3 -

- Question 4 -

- Question 5 -

Transcript – Nathan's Second Session – Skin Rash Resolved!

Out 8:10pm

In <u>7:10pm</u>
1: hr

Prior to the session, Nathan's father explained to me that there was no improvement.

Nathan would still not do it when asked to put on a shirt. I then asked him if he remembered me suggesting to him to back off, and to completely ignore the shirt "thing" He said then Nathan's mother would not be able to just leave Nathan alone about what he was wearing!

However, Nathan was wearing a brand new T-shirt, and reported to me feeling much, much better in his skin, although "it" was still there.

So I made him put the parts I wanted him to get in touch with in his hands to make Nathan aware of what he was using it for. The "What is so nice about it"

Part not comfortable	*Part comfortable in his skin*
- Stay by himself - Have a shirt routine he wants - Not to worry about fads - Always something (conflict) to think about - Keep his mind focused on shirts	- Being able to put on any shirt - Going to school, feeling comfortable - Putting a shirt on to go to a restaurant

<u>Resists "HAS TO' Innate stubbornness.</u>

Transcript Of Nathan's Second Session

Anny: I would like to know. You remember that I will touch your knees. You know that?

Nathan: Umh hum.

Anny: So just relax. Put your head back. Do you want a cushion?

Nathan: No it is okay.

Anny: It is okay.

So what I would like to know, is what happened since you came here? Anything improved, anything did not improve? Was there a difference? Did you feel different about yourself?

I have no idea.

Nathan: Well, I got this shirt.

Anny: You did?

Nathan: Yah, and I started wearing it so.

Anny: And you start what?

Nathan: I started wearing it and it does not really feel bad or anything like that.

Anny: It felt okay?

Nathan: Yup.

Anny: Okay. Very good.

Nathan: Remarkably like my other shirt, though, hey. Just without the holes.

Anny: I think it looks much better.

Nathan: Of course, it is not all torn up, hey.

Anny: No no, it is so. Okay, how do you feel that you could.
Now first of all, who bought that shirt?

Nathan: My Mom.

Anny: She did.

Nathan: Yup.

Anny: Okay. Were you with her when she bought it?

Nathan: No, she just brought it home and… .

Anny: She brought it home and you felt okay with it?

Nathan: Yup.

Anny: Okay very good. What is about it that you felt okay with it immediately?

Nathan: I do not know, I put it on and it was okay.

Anny: It was okay.

Nathan: Yah. Every time my Mom brings home one, she tells me to put it on and tell me what it feels like. And tell her what it feels like, I mean. And this one felt okay, which is different than the other ones of course, or else I would not be wearing it here.

Anny: All right. Very good. Anything else that made a difference?

Nathan: What do you mean?

Anny: Yah, umh. I do not know because I do not know your routine about other shirts.

Nathan: Well, when I was at school I noticed that the shirt that I usually wear to school, it felt better too. It did not feel quite as bad as it used to.

Anny: Okay, so there is an improvement?

Nathan: Yup.

Anny: So you are starting to feel better in your skin.

Nathan: Yah.

Anny: You find that funny do you?

Nathan: Yah.

Anny: Yah.

Nathan: Yah.

Anny: Yah. So, what can I do for you today. What would you like more of today? How does it feel to be able to wear something and be comfortable with it?

Nathan: It is pretty good actually. I wish I could do this with all the shirts. I tried to put on other shirts with just my bare skin, but it is still not entirely gone or something like that.

Anny: But there is an improvement?

Nathan: Yah.

Okay, very good.

Now, I am going to do something a little different today. It is still, it is still having access to your subconscious mind. Because you see, what I do here is making you aware of what is going on in your subconscious mind. That is all what I do.

And for me, my goal is for you to know what is going on inside of you.

Nathan: Okay.

Anny: And once you know what is going on inside of you, you will really do what you want with it. Because it is not for me to tell you what to do because it is your life. Your skin, your body. Okay?

Nathan: Okay.

Anny: So myself I am not going to tell you okay do it that way. No, no. What I want you to do is knowing what is going on inside of you and you know, many times it is pretty funny.

Nathan: It is what?

Anny: Funny.

Nathan: Ohh.

Anny: Many times, it is quite funny.

Nathan: Okay.

Anny: So be prepared for good laughs.

Nathan: Okay.

Anny: Okay.

Nathan: Okay.

Anny: All right. Now I know I have an accent Nathan and I know you noticed.

Nathan: Yah.

Anny: If you do not understand me, please say so.

Nathan: Okay.

Anny: Because then I can say it in a different way. Okay.

Nathan: All right.

Anny: All right.

So just relax there.

Just put your head back and become aware of your lungs, your lungs, just pay attention to your lungs. They are expanding and contracting. Expanding and contracting in a beautiful rhythmic manner. And every breathe that you take makes you go deeper and deeper and deeper into relaxation and as your breathe flows, as it comes, as it goes, notice that the sensation is a little cooler when you breathe in than when you breathe out. Just a little cooler. Just a little cooler. Just a little cooler.

And as you noticed that this sensation is a little cooler when you breathe in than when you breathe out, you become more and more relaxed. More and more relaxed. That right. More and more relaxed.

And you let all your cares fade away, fade away, fade away and you become so relaxed, so comfortable and become more and more aware of yourself. More and more aware of how you feel deep inside.

That is right. More and more and more and more relaxed. Letting all of your cares fade away, fade away, fade away, fade away and now as I am moving your hands, by taking your hands by the wrist, you become more and more relaxed, more and more comfortable.

That is right. And now Nathan, I would like you, in your mind, to put the part of you who does not feel comfortable with some shirts, let that part of you come in one of your hands and when it is there, simply turn up your hand so that I know that you are holding that part of you was not comfortable with some shirts. Let that part of you come in one of your hands and turn up your hand so I know you are holding it.

Thank you. Now, in the other hand, put the part of you who wants to feel comfortable in your skin. Yah, you want to be comfortable in your skin. That is right. So now, realizing though, that there are some things that we are not comfortable with and it happens to all of us. But let us say that that is the part of you - you know, that is quite reasonable and wants to be quite comfortable in your skin.

All right, so I am going to ask the part of you who wants to be comfortable in your skin to explain to the part of you who is not comfortable with lots of shirts. You know, different shirts. I would like the part of you who wants to be comfortable in your skin to explain to that part here what is nice about being comfortable in one's skin and I would like to hear it.

Nathan: Well, it will not hurt you anymore. It will not hurt me an more.

Anny: What is the positive side of that? Because you are mentioning hurt.

Nathan: Umh. Ohh. The positive side would be that I do not have to deal with it anymore.

Anny: So you are talking about dealing again.

Nathan: I do not have to worry about the ..

Anny: So your part is talking about the problem and I would like to know what is nice about it?

Nathan: In the morning I will not have to go around looking around for this certain shirt for school.

Anny: So, what would you do then if you did not have to do it?

Nathan: I do not have to look for my shirt.

Anny: Umh hum.

Nathan: I would be able to put on any shirt I want to.

Anny: So being able to put on any shirt you want. Okay. Anything else?

Nathan: I will be able to go to school and feel comfortable and everything.

Anny: Okay, going to school and feel comfortable. Now, what is about school that you are not comfortable in your skin usually?

Nathan: What is it about school?

Anny: Yah, because you say going to school and feel comfortable. So what is going on about school that you do not feel comfortable in your skin?

Nathan: I am not sure, it is everywhere. It might have started in school and I am not sure, I am not sure if that's ..

Anny: So what happens when you do not feel comfortable in a place?

Nathan: I get self-conscious because I usually stoop forward when I wear this shirt and I think I look pretty weird when I do that.

Anny: Okay. All right. So going to school and feel comfortable. Um hum.

Can you close your eyes and see yourself at school really comfortable?

Because it is that part here who is explaining it all and also see yourself in the morning able to put any shirt you want. Looking at your closet and just putting on what you like.

So ask that part to tell more about that part about what is nice about being comfortable in your skin. Go ahead.

Nathan: Ahh. I will not have to miss out on going to restaurants and stuff.

Anny: Okay. Good. All right. Okay, anything else?

Nathan: Umh.

Anny: So each time you tell me there, then close your eyes and see it. See it in your mind's eye. And then what comes next? What is nice about feeling comfortable in one's skin?

Nathan: People will not mention that I wear the same few shirts every day.

Anny: You do?

Nathan: Umh. Yah, usually actually my friend does. They usually drop it after awhile, but.

Anny: Okay, what would friends do then?

Nathan: Usually my friend would just - not my friend - not just my one friend - Brendon actually usually mentions it a lot. But usually once he says it, he will just drop it after awhile, so.

Anny: But, so what would happen if it feels good in your skin and it does not matter any more? They do not mention it anything any more.

Nathan: Right, they would eventually.

Anny: You will not be noticed anymore either, hey?

Nathan: I would not be noticed anymore? Well.

Anny: Nathan, I am doing this for a long time you know.

Nathan: Umh hum.

Anny: Umh hum.

Nathan: Yah. Well uhh. Noticed for what, noticed for that - for my shirts?

Anny: I have no idea. All what I say is that they will not notice you anymore, hey? How would that feel?

Nathan: That would feel better. I would not want to be noticed for something bad, but just like a few shirts every day. Yah. I am pretty sure they would notice me anyway, so.

Anny: So, would it still torture you if they have nothing to tell you?

Nathan: Umhhh.

Anny: Think about it.

Nathan: Will my friends still talk to me?

Anny: Well your friends, yes, but I am talking about other people.

Nathan: The other people usually do not mention my shirts at all. Yah, so. It is actually the people that I know really well that want to talk to me about my shirts, but the other people I talk to and they really will not mention it.

Anny: Okay, what will they talk about then? If they do not talk about your shirts?

Nathan: Just stuff. Stuff about school. They are not really close friends, so there is not much to talk about.

Anny: They are more acquaintances?

Nathan: Right, yah. So, usually just school.

Anny: By the sound of it. It is quite a conversation piece, huh?

Nathan: Yah, well.

Anny: Hum hum hum hum (laughing).

Nathan: It just (laughing) - usually just assorted stuff.

Anny: Umh hum. Okay, I am making you think, am I?

Nathan: Yah.

Anny: I told you, I am doing this for a long time.

Nathan: Yah.

Anny: And we have quite a way of entertaining ourselves. Um hum. I know you do not like it, okay. I know that. The thing is…

Okay, so ask that part anything else that would be nice to explain to that part. Anything else that would be nice if you were comfortable in your skin?

Nathan: I am worried about what I am supposed to say.

Anny: No. The only thing you are supposed to say is the truth according to you.

Nathan: Okay. So, what else did we miss. Well, I have already said I would not have to deal with the pain or what I would have to deal with just looking for the one shirt. Umh. Umh. Okay. I guess that there would be. Hum.

You would not be noticed anymore either, huh?

Nathan: Oh, I would be noticed. I would just uhh. I am pretty funny at school so.

Anny: Are you?

Nathan: Yup. So, I would be noticed for that, just not my shirts.

Anny: Okay.

Okay. Now, each part has it's time at talking. I would like that part of you here that does not feel comfortable to tell that part here what is so nice about not feeling comfortable. What is nice about it?

Nathan: I can stay by myself.

Anny: What?

Nathan: I can stay by myself without really worrying about.

Anny: Okay. Go ahead because I do not know, it is you not me. So I really want you to just think about it. What is nice and let that part really make you aware of some stuff.

Nathan: I have a routine. If I am uncomfortable. I just wear the few shirts instead of having to switch around the holly shirts.

Anny: So you have a routine.

Nathan: Um hum. I do not have to worry about fads or anything like that.

Anny: Okay, just a moment. You have a shirt routine really.

Nathan: Right.

Anny: And what do you not have to worry with?

Nathan: I would not have to worry about fads or anything like that.

Anny: That is a very good point. I never thought about it, but you are right. Anything else? Just go ahead. Just get in touch with that part of you.

Nathan: It would always be something to think about.

Anny: What are you supposed to think about? What is it? What is it?

Nathan: I do not know, it would always be something to have to worry about. It would be some kind of conflict.

Anny: Okay, always something of a conflict.

Nathan: That does not seem like a very good reason though.

Anny: No, you would be surprised. There is a lot of stuff here. Okay, go ahead.

Nathan: I think that is it.

Anny: You would be by yourself. You have a shirt thing. You have to not worry about fads. And I never thought about it, but are you ever right there. And always something to think about, yah. When you think about that, you do not have to think about anything else either, huh. So it keeps your mind occupied. Is that correct?

Nathan: Well, when I am wearing a shirt anyway, it keeps my mind occupied. I do not always think about it, like just sitting there and thinking about shirts, but when I am wearing it, it is always something.

When you what?

Nathan: When I am wearing a shirt, it is always, I am always thinking about it. Rather than concentrating on something that I am supposed to be concentrating on.

Anny: So it keeps your mind focussed on shirts.

Nathan: Right. Umh.

Anny: Okay, very good. Anything else?

Nathan: No.

Anny: Now, I m going to ask that part to ask that part if you did not have to think about shirts all the time, what would happen then?

Nathan: I would probably get better marks in school.

Anny: Ha ha ha ha (laughing).

Nathan: I have already got pretty good marks in school, but I am sure I could get better. I actually really started even thinking about shirts some more in Junior High and my marks kinda dropped off a bit by then. I was an honour student in Elementary and it dropped off to more like a semi-honours. Like honourable mention is what it is called.

Anny: I am going to ask you just close your eyes for a minute and see your shirts in your closets. Whatever you see if fine with me and ask yourself, what is it about you, a bright young man, that gives so much power to shirts?

Because you are bright, quite intelligent. I think you have a good sense of humour and what is it about a bright young man like you that gives so much power to a shirt? That has no brains, no nothing?

Nathan: I never thought about it that way. Yah. It does not make sense that I would make that rule my day, pretty much.

Anny: You let it run your life.

Nathan: Yah, whenever I wear it, it is what. Yah. So what.

Anny: So I would like you to go inside and ask that inside of you to make you aware of something.

There is something about it. There is something about it and go inside of you and ask that part of you what can be improved now inside of you so that you can just put a shirt where it belongs. Just something there that is hanging in the closet. You can wear it or not wear it. It has no intelligence of it's own. It cannot do anything by itself. So go inside of you Nathan, go inside and ask that part of you there. Ask that part of you to make you aware of something about it. Something about it.

Nathan: Umh. Clothes are a real important aspect of the day, hey. Everyone wears them of course.

Anny: Well yah, because otherwise you would end up exposed.

Nathan: So, that might even be the reason why I do not like them. You always have to wear them. So.

Anny: Yes, but you can. Ah huh. Can you repeat that again, that is a pretty good thing that you just told me.

Nathan: Everybody wears them and you always have to wear them all the time. So.

Anny: And how do you feel about something that you have to. Deep down. Deep, deep down.

Nathan: Well, if I have to do it, I usually do not like to do it.

Anny: Ha ha ha ha (laughing).

Nathan: The same thing with pretty much everything else. If my parents tell me I have to do it, I hate it. I just do not do it.

Anny: Okay. All right. So, all right. We are getting somewhere here. So I am going to ask you to go inside of you and ask that part of you, what can you do to improve that part that feels that way about anything really.

Nathan: Well, I can become less stubborn. I can be less stubborn about it. That actually may even be it because everything that my parents tell me that I have to learn to do, or else there will be problems and stuff, I usually do not try to learn it. Like this may seem stupid, but when I…

Anny: No, no, everything you say is very intelligent I can tell you, so tell me.

Nathan: Well, when I played hockey, I never stopped on my left foot. I had learned to stop on my right foot, but I had stopped on my left foot and I knew that I had to, but my Dad told me that I have to and I never really tried to do it. I am not sure whether it was actually because of that or if it was an actual problem. I did try to stop on the left foot before, but it did not really work out that well, so.

Anny: Yah. I understand that very well. What I wonder is how come… well I do not know anything about hockey and I do not know how to skate because I come from Africa and I never saw ice before I came to Canada so. So, but okay anything else that is like that, when you are told that you have to, that you are making a point of nothing?

Nathan: Oh, my Dad can give you a whole list about it, but I cannot really remember anything.

Anny: Okay, and all right. And you do not like that, huh?

Nathan: Yah. It will….

Anny: There is a part of you who puts the brakes on, huh?

Nathan: Right.

Anny: Can you go inside, go inside that part here who really likes not to be comfortable. Ask that part, go inside that part that does not like to be comfortable for all kind of reasons.

About shirts, how old are you in that thing about you have to wear it, well I will not. How old is Nathan?

Nathan: How long have I been like that do you mean?

Anny: Go inside the feeling, okay.
I am going to explain it slowly. There is a part of you who does not want to wear all kind of shirts. Right?

Nathan: Right.

Anny: Okay, connect with that part of you that is deep down inside and ask that part what was the idea, the decision. What was it that made you decide no, I will not wear what I have to wear.

Go inside, go inside. Feel that feeling.

Nathan: Umh. I do not know. It is like it just happened one day. It is so long ago when this started, I cannot even remember how it started, so.

Anny: The feeling remembers. Remembers everything. But for that you have to really connect with it. So I am going to help you with that.

Stare at my fingers. Listen to my voice. Keep your gaze on my fingers and listen to my voice. Keep your gaze on my fingers. Take a deep breathe Nathan and as you exhale close your eyes and become more and more aware of something about having to wear it. So it is not a choice. You were told here it is, you wear it.

And as I am repeating that, you are going to have feelings, a feeling is coming from inside of you. A feeling, a feeling, a feeling, a feeling. And what is it and trust whatever awareness comes to you. Just trust it.

Nathan: Okay, the first day I was going to school I was told by my Mom that I have to wear something nice on the first day of school. I probably did not like that because the word have to came up again.

Anny: Ah huh. It is the have to.

Nathan: Yah.

Anny: Do you have pictures of you when you were the little boy like that?

Nathan: Yah, somewhere. My Mom does.

Anny: Do you remember how they looked like? How you looked like as a little boy?

Nathan: No. No, I do not have any pictures really.

Anny: You do not remember. Can you check inside to see if you can be able to just check to know if you feel like that little boy who was told he has to?

Nathan: I cannot imagine a six year old being really upset about that.

Anny: Yah.

Nathan: Well, yah but I know but ah. Like really understanding whether it is....

Anny: Well, I am pretty sure it was not the first time neither.

Nathan: Probably, of course. But yah, maybe because I had to wear shirts I started to dislike them and after awhile that just turned into pain or something like that.

Anny: I would like you to connect with that kid inside of you. Just close your eyes and connect with it. And tell me if you can do it?

Connect with that feeling inside. Ah hum, I have to do it. Even now. Feeling inside if you are told you have to do it and how does it feel inside when you are told you have to do it. How does that feel Nathan? Even now. How does it feel when you have to do it?

Nathan: Cannot really match a word with how it feels because it really is not anger or upset or anything but.

Anny: Okay. That is all right.

Nathan: It is like just an innate stubbornness.

Anny: Okay, very good. Excellent. Innate stubbornness. Okay. I am going to ask that innate stubbornness of yours there to look at you now. Here you are 15 years old and how about starting to wear things so that it is nice for others to look at you. And it is your choice. I am going to explain to you how come I am saying that. There are nice cars and ragged cars, right. Which one do you like to look at?

Nathan: Well the nice car of course.

Anny: Of course. It is the same when you look at someone. You know it is very pleasant when someone wears something nice. It is nice to look at. So how about starting to choose to wear things so it is pleasant to look at. Pleasant can be something as simple as the right color for you. Just like what you wear today goes very well with the color of your skin. It can be just something like that. It does not have to be - you know, designer jeans, things like that. I am not talking about that. I am talking about having a knack at wearing something that is pleasant to look at. It has nothing to do with fad. How would you like that?

Nathan: Yah, I guess I would like that. To wear a shirt that looks nice and not be bothered by it or anything.

Anny: Yah, and feels good for you. Because you know I suppose you like homey things.

Nathan: I like which?

Anny: Homey.

Nathan: Well yah.

Anny: Comfortable.

Nathan: Right.

Anny: You look like a young man that likes to wear something that is comfortable. Okay, is there anything that you can do inside to say that I am 15 years old now. I can choose to wear what I want, instead of my skin telling me yes or no.

Nathan: Um hum.

Anny: Have a look at your closet and the shirts. In your mind, go to your closet and see the shirts. And notice how much power you give those things. Occupying your mind all the time. Just a piece of rag that hangs there. Anything you can do so that you are the boss instead of the shirts.

Nathan: Ahh, yah. Well I do not know what I could do, or else I would have done it by now.

Anny: You are right. What are they?

Nathan: Yah, this. I do not want to have this problem any more so this.

Anny: You have had enough of it, huh?

Nathan: Right, this stubbornness about shirts is kinda going against my stubbornness. I am letting shirts dictate what I do, so, yah. It is a little weird.

Anny: Did you learn something about you today?

Nathan: Yah. I am nuts.

Anny: Humm?

Nathan: I am nuts, but yah. No, I am just kidding, but I guess my Dad is right, I am really stubborn, but.

Anny: Yah, but you change this - who is the boss?

Nathan: When it comes to the shirts? I guess the shirts will be the boss because I am not really in charge.

Anny: Yah, you are not really in charge really.

A technique I believe is called time line.

So, okay. You know when it **started**. You likely were told you have to wear that and it could be even done before you going to school.

And you are not going to like that at all, but then you do not like anything that you have to do.

Nathan: Well, what I am told that I have to do anyway.

Anny: Okay, you know when you have to do it.

Nathan: But.

Anny: When you are told you have to do it.

Nathan: Right, I do not like that.

Anny: Okay, very good. So you know when it started. It started with whatever. There is something interesting about this shirt though. Who did you argue the most about shirts? Who do you argue with?

Nathan: My Mom because my Mom sends us off to school and that is when the problem comes.

Anny: Okay. All right. So anyway. You know when it **started.** You do not know exactly when, but you have a good idea.

Now you know when it was the **worst** that it got to really become a problem?

Nathan: Grade 7.

Anny: Grade 7.

Nathan: Yup.

Anny: Okay. That is Junior High. Because I am not from here, so I have to think. Okay Junior High.

All right. Now, so you know when it **started.** You know the **middle** where it was the worst and now in your mind advance to when it is completely **gone**. Wherever that is. Your decision and I do not want to know it. I really do not want to know because that is none of my business. You go there. When is it going to end? Now when you got it, let me know. When do you want it to end?

Nathan: When do I want this to end. Well, I have got that.

Anny: Okay, very good. All right. Do it again.

You know the beginning.
You know the middle.
Now you go to the end of it.

And how does that feel.

Nathan: The end. That feels good. I want to get over this.

Anny: Okay.

Nathan: I have had enough of it. It has been way too long. For anything, it is been way too long. Even if it was…

Anny: It became outdated.

Nathan: Yah, it is become stale. It is just too old now.

Anny: Okay, so as you are at the end there, have a look at how you feel in the shirt that you are wearing today and how does that feel? Feels okay huh?

Nathan: Feels which?

Anny: Okay.

Nathan: Yah.

Anny: Yah. Um hum.

Nathan: Which is odd because this was bought new. It was not bought second hand or anything, so.

Anny: So that is a very pretty huge improvement.

So now look at your closet and say hum - that looks good to me today. Wear it and feel comfortable with it. In your mind.

And do it all over and over again.

Other shirts. Another day, have a look into that closet. Hum. What do you feel like wearing that day? Choose what you want and notice how it feels inside to be able to choose what you want.

There is something inside of you that is shifting and deep inside of you there is a part of you who is making all the necessary improvements right now so that you can be the boss now. You are the boss. Feeling great in every way. You are the boss. You are the one who chooses, feeling great in every way. How do you feel now?

Nathan: Very good. I do not have to worry about anything, and I am in charge of it all.

Anny: Anything else that you feel will make you more in charge of it all?

Nathan: Like what do you mean?

Anny: I have no idea, just because I do not know the routine at home and so forth. What do you feel would make you really in charge of that skin of yours really? Feeling good in your skin and it is your choice.

Nathan: If my parents just left me alone about it.

Anny: Okay. All right.

Nathan: If they did not mention anything about it. It is like. If they did not mind me even going to school in ratty clothes after awhile, I think it would start to go away or something. Because. .

Anny: You know what, I think you are right. Okay. I think you are right. Yah. So, anything else today. What do you feel about this session today? Did you learn something about yourself?

Nathan: Yah. Actually.

Anny: I told you it would be funny. Ha ha ha (laughing).

Nathan: Gheez, I am stubborn. Ha ha ha.

Anny: Yah, you are.

Nathan: Yah, oh man.

Anny: I told you it is funny.

Nathan: Well, yah I think it would actually help. Like if I was headed off to school and my Mom did not say anything about what I was wearing, about what I was going to wear when I went there. I think it would help. Because I cannot imagine other people, other people's moms saying every day that you are supposed to wear this and that because from the stuff that the kids wear at school, I cannot think that their parents would want them to know they are like that, but. Yah.

Anny: Okay, very good. Um hum. All right, I am thinking about something and I am smiling. I am going to finish your session, but before that I would like you to just relax. And I would like you to imagine you are 45. Yah, that is 30 years from now, right?

Nathan: Yah.

Anny: And here you are. You have your own kids and you show them pictures of you with those shirts and how do you feel? As you look back and how stubborn you were about making your points with those shirts. How will you look at it?

Nathan: I actually think I would be embarrassed.

Anny: Would you?

Nathan: Yah.

Anny: I think I would laugh so hard. I would have a tummy ache.

Nathan: I am not sure if I would really laugh.

Anny: I think it is funny.

Nathan: Well, I wear some pretty atrocious things. Well…

Anny: That is all right. Some kids - you told me yourself, some kids wear some pretty atrocious things too.

Nathan: Yah but. Yah, I guess it would be pretty funny.

Anny: Yah, and your kids looking at that would say, that was you Dad. My God.

Nathan: My God you were insane. Ha ha, but yah.

Anny: And if your kids are as smart as you, they would say, well so Dad do not tell me what to do, look at you. Ha ha ha ha (laughing).

Nathan: Ha ha - I hope they are as smart as me, but yah.

Anny: You will find that young people are very smart. Much smarter than people give them credit for.

Okay, anything else I can do to help you? Think about it.

Nathan: Well, I am not really sure. God I have real troubles having to pull things out of the hat. I can probably think of lots of other things when I am….

Anny: You did not expect me to ask you that.

Nathan: Right, yah.

Anny: I explained that to you at the beginning of the session.

Remember something Nathan, my goal is for you to know what you are doing and you make a decision of what to do with it because it is your life, your skin. Your stubbornness and it is like that for everybody here. I want them to know what they are doing. What games they are playing.

Nathan: But the problem is yah.

Anny: Yah you can call it a problem, but I do not call it a problem.

Nathan: Well, that is what it is. It is got to be fixed, it is a problem.

Anny: Yup, okay remember what Shakespeare said, we are all actors and the world is stage. Okay. Anything else. That is it for today.

Nathan: Yah I guess.

Anny: Very good. I am going to stop the recording.

At the end of the session, when alone with Nathan's father, I explained it was important to back off and stop mentioning clothes.

Nathan's father explained they (Nathan's Mother and him) had to keep telling what to do, otherwise, Nathan would do nothing, just sit there.

I do not remember exactly how the conversation went. All I remember is, at one point, Nathan's father mention it was important to keep Nathan under control and tell him what to do.

And I replied: "Right, and no matter what you do, you cannot tell him what to wear."
Nathan's father was speechless for a good minute.

Then, I suggested they give Nathan the money they budget for his clothes, and tell him to buy his own and to be very firm in the allowance. If he runs out of money, well, tough. Be firm on that.

Nathan's father thought a little, and said, yes, they would do that.

Questions About Jenney's Session

- Question 1 -
- Question 2 -
- Question 3 -
- Question 4 -
- Question 5 -

Transcript – Jenney (17 Years Old) – Memory Loss

Following A Car Accident

Note: Her mother had taken HYP 101 several years prior to come here.

Anny: Now before we do anything. I know you experience hypnosis because of your Mother and I am very pleased. I am quite impressed as a matter of fact. I am pleased. Now I have learned through the years that when I use a technique called anchoring during hypnotherapy session, the session is faster, smoother, much more comfortable and we come to a resolution much, much faster. That technique of anchoring can be done in many, many ways and the way I do it, I will be touching your knees and it will be a firm touch like that. Sometimes I will touch this knee. Sometimes the other. Sometimes both and I would like to have your permission to do so.

Jenney: Yes.

Anny: Okay. Thank you. Now I understand you are in school.

Jenney: Yes.

Anny: What grade are you in.

Jenney: Grade 12.

Anny: You are in grade 12.

Jenney: Yes.

Anny: Grade 12. All right. And so when are you finished?

Jenney: June.

Anny: In June.

Jenney: Yes.

Anny: Okay you graduate

Jenney: In June.

Anny: In June.

Jenney: 2009.

Anny: What ?

Jenney: 2009

Anny: Yah, 2009. Now what are you planning to do after that? What are your plans so far?

Jenney: Well, I do not know. Before the accident I wanted to go to med school.

Anny: You what?

Jenney: I wanted to go to med school.

Anny: Yes, and?

Jenney: And now my grades have dropped like 20% in every class. I went from like 90's and 80's to like 60's and 50's.

Anny: Yah, but that is since when did they drop?

Jenney: A month ago.

Anny: Oh, since the accident, well that is temporary. What do you want to do?

Jenney: I want to go to med school.

Anny: You want to go to med school.

Jenney: Yah.

Anny: Okay. Since when did you want to do that?

Jenney: Since I was about 3 years old.

Anny: Is that right? What is it about it that med school has such an attraction to you?

Jenney: I do not know, helping people and I do not know, I just want to help people. Cause I really do not care about the money, it is just the fact that I can like save somebody's life.

Anny: You know what, that is true.

Jenney: Umm humm. I could save like so many people's lives in just one day.

Anny: Which is true.

Jenney: And doctors do not get enough credit.

Anny: That is true too. Okay, since 3 years old uhh. All right. I think that is great.

Jenney: (Clearing throat)

Anny: Anything in particular that you remember that this made you decide that you wanted to go to med school?

Jenney: Yah, my Mom used to take me to work with her all the time.

Anny: Yes.

Jenney: When I was little and I used to see doctors and actually I used to go look at the babies all the time.

Anny: Did you?

Jenney: Yah, through like you know the nursery or whatever.

Anny: Umm humm.

Jenney: And, I decided that some day I might want to deliver babies or be a paediatrician. And that is why I wanted to be a doctor.

Anny: Okay. I would like you to do something.

Jenney: Yes.

Anny: Now, about two months ago you could see yourself as a paediatrician.

Jenney: Ohh yahh.

Anny: Close your eyes and see yourself there. See yourself as a very good paediatrician truly enjoying your work, having a passion for it and there is something I would like you to do from now on. Each time you do not feel things are going the way they should, get that image back and then become aware of that light inside of you. The spark of life that you have inside of you. Become aware of that, just connect with it. It is like a mini sun in your chest and tell that light of yours, that spark of life that that is what you want. You want to be fine. That is what you want. And you know what, trust that light inside of you. Trust it. The thing is you have to send it that message all the time. That is what I want. And how it is going to happen, trust that light. Do you know what I discovered the other day? There was a scientist who came here.

Jenney: Ummm humm.

Anny: I really do not remember for what anymore, because I see a lot of people here, but I know she was a scientist and we got to talk. Do you know that they still do not know what gives life?

Jenney: Really.

Anny: That is a mystery. They know the eggs and sperms and all that.

Jenney: Well yah, that is (huh huh huh).

Anny: But they do not know

Jenney: What makes life…

Anny: Yah.

Jenney: What makes that happen. What makes us live.

Anny: Yes.

Jenney: What makes animals live?

Anny: How come…

Jenney: That is something I wondered my entire life.

Anny: And then I said to her, so you tell me that in 2009, they still do not know how a seed turns out as a radish. She said no. So, I knew the mystery is in that light inside of you, so trust it. Totally trust it.

Jenney: That is cool.

Anny: Totally trust it and send it the image of what you want. What do you want? What do you want? And especially the days you feel down, get that image and give it to that light.

Jenney: And hold on to it.

Anny: That is what I want. Imagine yourself holding a picture of you as you are doing your work and you can see yourself, you know, with your lab coat or whatever you are going to wear, you know, doing your work. And keep that in mind. And because there is a mystery within all of us and it is that energy that gives life. So, I would like you to …

Jenney: (sneeze)

Anny: Understand that it is that light that heals everything. You have to trust it though. You have to trust it. So just see yourself there. Know you will be fine. After all, that accident happened only a month ago and when one looks at you, you would never know. I understand you were injured and everything.

Jenney: Umm humm.

Anny: You would never know. So there is something inside there that is repairing everything.

Jenney: That is true.

Anny: Yah, and it will repair your memory.

Jenney: The doctors could not believe how fast my head healed.

Anny: You see.

Jenney: Like on the outside.

Anny: Oh yah. And it will, hey.

Jenney: So maybe it is healing just as fast on the inside.

Anny: Umm humm. Umm humm. Okay. I am going to do something and I want to check it out. It is because I am going to use several techniques.

Jenney: Umm humm.

Anny: Because of the situation. You know, having been in an accident like that. I am going to….

All right, you will tell me if it is comfortable because you, you know, is it comfortable when I hold your head like that?

Jenney: Umm humm.

Emotional Stress Release:

Anny: Okay, I would like you to tell me what happened? What happened? Tell me the whole thing.

Jenney: In the accident?

Anny: Yes.

Jenney: We were driving to my friend's house.

Anny: To what?

Jenney: To my friend's house.

Anny: Okay.

Jenney: I was going to go to a movie. And we were turning left on 157th and St. Albert Trail and then next thing you know I saw a car coming towards us and I totally blacked out.

Anny: Is that right?

Jenney: Yah.

Anny: And then what happened next?

Jenney: And the next thing you know the ambulance and everybody was there and I saw my Dad standing outside the car and we were trying to get my Mom from the other side. And she was trying to say something to me. I do not know. And the next thing you know I was in the ambulance on a stretcher.

Anny: And then what happened?

Jenney: They were asking me what my name was (clear throat) and I did not know. So they told me my name was Jenney and then they asked me like 5 minutes later what my name was and I still did not know.

Anny: Okay. How do you remember that, that they asked you that?

Jenney: I do not know.

Anny: Okay, you remember that though.

Jenney: (laughter)

Anny: Okay.

Jenney: And then I was in the hospital.

Anny: Umm humm.

Jenney: And like waiting by the emergency.

Anny: Umm humm.

Jenney: And then the next thing you know. Like, I do not know I kept having like black outs.

Anny: Umm humm. Of course you did.

Jenney: Then I was in the emergency room and they had me strapped down to the stretcher still. And I felt like sharp, sharp pains in the back of my head.

Anny: Umm humm.

Jenney: And they kept telling me it was fine and I was kinda getting angry with them because I was like no it really hurts. Huh.

Anny: Of course.

Jenney: And they had me there for like two hours without doing anything. They just kept talking to me and stuff. Cause they were trying to work on my Mom to make sure she was alive and stuff and so they took like they unstrapped me after they did my stitches and stuff.

Anny: Umm humm.

Jenney: And it was bobby pins sticking into the back of my head.

Anny: Umm humm.

Jenney: And then I went to the bathroom to clean my face.

Anny: You did?

Jenney: And there was blood all over down my shirt and all over my jacket and everywhere.

Anny: Yah, a head really bleeds a lot, huh.

Jenney: When, when before the accident, when I saw the car coming, I covered my face with my jacket.

Anny: You did? With your jacket?

Jenney: Yah. So I did not. That is why my face is not like messed up.

Anny: That was a very good response, huh.

Jenney: Yah, I know and I do not even know why I did. Actually, there is another thing I remember. Two minutes before the accident, I was sitting by the window seat and for some unknown reason, I moved to the middle. I do not even know why I did it.

Anny: Okay.

Jenney: But if I would have stayed there, I might have been dead.

Anny: Umm humm.

Jenney: Because I would have hit my head a lot harder on that window and it might have killed me. For some unknown reason, I moved to the middle seat.

Anny: It was that light inside of you.

Jenney: Umm humm. And then, when I was in the bathroom cleaning my face and stuff.

Anny: Umm humm.

Jenney: I realized that I had two really big cuts on my head and they did not do anything with that.

Anny: They did not do it?

Jenney: No, and I like lifted the skin and I could see my skull.

Anny: How does that look like?

Jenney: Unbelievably disgusting.

Anny: Is that right? (laughter)

Jenney: (laughter)

Anny: I find it very interesting because….

Jenney: I could like see the bone and….

Anny: Yes, you do. I find that fascinating because I saw it once too on someone else though. And you can see the bones and everything.

Jenney: Yah.

Anny: Yah.

Jenney: And there was like, like really nasty. Huh. So I went back and there was more blood with this.

Anny: Of course.

Jenney: I lifted the skin and it …

Anny: It was cleansing itself, huh?

Jenney: Yup. So then they stitched that up and I went and made sure my Mom was okay, but I kept having dizzy spells.

Anny: Of course you did.

Jenney: And I could not stand up.

Anny: Umm humm.

Jenney: And ever since my memory as been really bad.

Anny: Is that right?

Jenney: And I have a hard time focussing.

Anny: All right. Take a deep breath and as you exhale, it is if though you know you are rewinding a video in your mind. Rewind everything to, I would like you to go to when you got into the car. Rewind everything, but this time you go further. And when you are, when you were getting into the car to go to your friend. That minute.

Jenney: Ummm humm.

Anny: When you are there, let me know.

Jenney: I went a little bit farther than that. I remember what happened

Anny: Okay, okay, just go ahead. Go further than that.

Jenney: Further than?

Anny: Whatever. Where did you go?

Jenney: I went back to school that day before I left.

Anny: Excellent. Okay, and then what happened next?

Jenney: My friend asked me.

Anny: Umm humm.

Jenney: If I wanted to go to Texas Chainsaw Massacre with her and Danny and I was all excited to go and I got on the bus and I was very happy.

Anny: Umm humm.

Jenney: And I was on my way home and I was talking to a friend of mine. Her name is Marla. About what she was going to do on the weekend.

Anny: Umm humm.

Jenney: And then I got home. What did I do. I had supper.

Anny: Umm humm.

Jenney: And Mom gave me money for the movie and for a treat and that is what I had in my pocket.

Anny: Okay.

Jenney: I had a ten-dollar bill and a loonie and two quarters and that is what made the big bruise on my leg.

Anny: Umm humm.

Jenney: And then I was gonna take the bus at five o'clock, but she did not call me. She did not call until almost six and when she called at six. But she was going to call me, but she took a nap instead.

Anny: (laughter)

Jenney: And so it was six o'clock and Mom and Dad were going out, so they gave me a ride instead of taking the bus. And we got into the car and we were on our way and we were talking about what time I was going to be home and stuff.

Anny: Umm humm.

Jenney: And the next thing you know, we were in the accident.

Anny: Okay, tell me the details again. I know it is not very pleasant, but just go ahead. Tell me again. And then what happened. So you got into the car and you were talking about what time you would get home and everything and then what happened next?

Jenney: And then, we were going to turn off 137th Street and St. Albert Trail and looked up and the light changed from yellow to red. I cannot remember which one was it. It was the one right in front of me or the one right beside me. But I looked over and I saw the car coming, so I covered my face and kinda leaned to my right, to my left.

Anny: Umm humm.

Jenney: And, the car hit. And like I heard a really loud noise. And the next thing you know, actually, I remember something else. Dad got out of the car and lifted up the back seat and he had paper towels and he gave them to me to wipe my face and I looked down at my hand and it was covered in blood. Cause I like had my hand over my face still.

Anny: Umm humm.

Jenney: Sometime during that, I must have – I do not think I let go of my head when I hit it. I do not think I let go of my face.

Anny: Okay, so he gave you some paper towels.

Jenney: Yup. He gave me some paper towels to clean off my face and then my Mom could not. Like she kept trying to ask me how I was.

Anny: Umm humm.

Jenney: And if I was okay, but she was having a hard time breathing. Because she has really bad asthma and the car when it hit her. Like it hit her door and moved it in two feet.

Anny: Umm humm.

Jenney: So it kinda collapsed her lungs, I guess. Umm, and then the ambulance came.

Anny: Umm humm.

Jenney: But the fire fighters came first to get Mom out of the car.

Anny: They did?

Jenney: I think so.

Anny: Okay, they are quite fast, huh?

Jenney: Yah.

Anny: Okay.

Jenney: And the police were there and we were on the news, but like we were not on the news, I think the accident was, or something.

Anny: Umm humm.

Jenney: I cannot. I really do not know. But it was on the news (clearing throat). And …

Anny: I would like you to tell me something?

Jenney: Uhh huhh.

Anny: The car that came towards you. What type of car? I know it was a split of a second, but.

Jenney: It was a greenish colour.

Anny: Okay.

Jenney: And I think it was a Chev.

Anny: Okay. And what happened

Jenney: It was four doors.

Anny: And what happened with the driver.

Jenney: Hummm?

Anny: The driver, what happened with that driver?

Jenney: I think he hit his head on the steering wheel.

Anny: What?

Jenney: I think he hit his head on the steering wheel or something.

Anny: Ummm humm.

Jenney: But I think I saw him and he was bleeding.

Anny: Okay. Well of course he was. Okay, so your Mother, the fire fighters came, got your Mother out of there, ambulance was there, you were on the news.

Jenney: I remember them strapping me down to the thing and trying to get me out of the car without moving me too much.

Anny: Umm humm.

Jenney: (clearing throat) And then taking me into the ambulance.

Anny: Okay.

Jenney: And they kept trying to ask me what my name was and trying to ask me questions. Trying to keep me conscious.

Anny: Ohhh yah.

Jenney: But I do not think. I do not know. I kept telling them that I did not know what they were talking about. Huh. (laughter)

Anny: (laughter)

Jenney: And then (laughter) they were like you have been in an accident. And I was like, no. I do not know what you are talking about (laughter) and I was in the entrance waiting to go into the emergency room and Mom was already in there.

Anny: Umm humm.

Jenney: Because they took her straight in because she was not breathing.

Anny: Umm humm.

Jenney: And I was in the emergency room right next to her. They were going to take me to the Sturgeon (clearing throat) and Mom to the Alex, but Mom told them that we would both have to be at the same hospital or I will freak out. (laughter)

Anny: Umm humm.

Jenney: So then I was in the emergency room and I was getting sharp pains in the back of my head and the nurses kept talking to me and telling me that I was going to be okay and telling me that I had head injuries and my ear was cut open, but that I would be fine. Uhh. They did stitches on my ear and took the bobby pins out of the back of my head.

Anny: The what?

Jenney: Because I thought it was glass. Bobby pins, because I thought it was glass sticking in the back of my head. And after they were done I tried, well actually first I tried to stand up and I had to lie back down because I was dizzy.

Anny: Of course you were.

Jenney: Huhh.

Anny: Of course you were.

Jenney: And then I ended up standing up and I went to the bathroom. I found it and I was cleaning the blood off my face and down my neck and stuff and I found two more cuts. Well gashes.

Anny: They did not even look at it, huh?

Jenney: No.

Anny: No, so what did they say when they saw it?

Jenney: They were like, oh well we better fix that. Huh, so they kinda.

Anny: You know what. I must say something, can I ask you to close your eyes. See the people who stitched you up and tell them how good a job they done because even when you know you were cut, you can see nothing, so they did a pretty good job. And when you are finished, say so. Now,

Jenney: Umm humm.

Anny: become aware of your light. The spark of life. It is like a mini sun in your chest and thank it for having repaired the outside that fast and in your mind, show them to go inside and repair it too. With the same expertise, the same know how and the same speed as the outside. Thank them for that in advance. And then you open your eyes. All right.

Jenney: Umm

Anny: So now I am going to ask you to rewind the movie of time again. All the way back to the day before when your friend asked if you wanted to go to that movie. And when you are back there, let me know.

Jenney: I am back to when my friend asked me to go to the movie.

Anny: All right. Now you are going to review everything again and stop here to when you saw the car and covered your face, okay.

Jenney: (clear throat) So you want me to tell you again?

Anny: And you tell me then.

Jenney: Do you want me to tell you again then?

Anny: No, you just go there and when you are there, let me know.

Jenney: I am there.

Anny: Now listen carefully. At the speed that I will move my hands where they are, go to the top of your head and bring them back where they are now. From where you stopped, you are going to go all the way to when they stitched you back completely, you know the face there and at the same time, from where you stopped, you are going to go back to when your friend asked you, what you are going to do to the next day, because she wanted you to join her. Are you understanding what I mean?

Jenney: Umm humm.

Anny: It is like stretching it.

Jenney: Say that again.

Anny: From where you stopped.

Jenney: Umm humm.

Anny: You are going to go all the way back to when your friend asked you.

Jenney: Umm humm.

Anny: And at the same time, from where you stopped, you are going to go all the way back to when they stitched you, the rest of you.

Jenney: Umm humm.

Anny: Okay, it is like stretching it. Okay.

Jenney: Umm humm.

Anny: Take a deep breath. (breathing in) and stretch it (breathing out slowly). And keep breathing. Keep breathing. Now, rewind everything to when your friend asked you the day before and when you are back there, here, let me know.

Jenney: Umm humm.

Anny: Now you review it again and stop again here. And when you are there, let me know. (pause) All right.

Jenney: Umm humm.

Anny: Now you are going to stretch it again. Okay, take a deep breath and as you exhale (breath out), stretch it. All right. How do you feel now?

End of Emotional Stress Release

Jenney: It does not hurt as much.

Anny: Is it not interesting. Yah, this is a special technique I learned for in cases like yours. Yah. So it feels better inside?

Jenney: I could remember a lot more of the accident. A lot more of what happened before the accident.

Anny: Oh yes, so you will find that your memory is fine. It is that I found that that technique is because the whatever happened was not easy to take and to experience, so it is like we put something over us, over our head to not remember the details.

Jenney: Umm humm.

Anny: But guess what? That technique lifts the hood.

Jenney: I almost remember perfectly.

Anny: I must say. Are you impressed?

Jenney: Yah.

Anny: Yahhh.

Jenney: Maybe I did not black out. Maybe I just made myself forget.

Anny: Whatever. What counts is that you know your memory is fine. It is simply for whatever reason and it is what happened there is totally normal you know that you because who wants to …

Jenney: (laugh)

Anny: You know…

Jenney: Who wants to remember it?

Anny: So, that is the special technique I learned for cases like yours. And you impressed yourself did you not? You have got a pretty good memory huh?

Jenney: Umm humm.

Anny: Umm humm.

Jenney: The last time I went over it, I remembered specific details of what happened that day. And specific things that I said and that other people said and that is the kind of stuff that I am having troubles remembering.

Anny: You see, how. And all of a sudden….

Jenney: That I was having a hard time.

Anny: Things are quite easy to remember. You surprised yourself, did you not?

Jenney: Yah.

Anny: Umm humm.

Jenney: Quite.

Anny: Yah. Everything is there and how does it feel inside now? Inside that head of yours, how does it feel?

Jenney: Better. But I still have pain right here.

Anny: Yah, well all right. You know, since you will be a doctor, you are going to learn something here. You will learn that there is something about us that is quite unique. It is a privilege to be a human being. By the way, I am very spiritual and I am not religious. But I learned something about life. Because when you do hypnosis, you touch the soul of the people, so I learned a lot. Yah, so. Uhh huhh, your memory is much better than you thought, huh?

Jenney: Uhhh huhh (laugh).

Anny: You find that funny do you? (laughter) How does that make you feel?

Jenney: Gives me maybe new hope that I may have lost in the last month (clearing throat).

Anny: How does that feel?

Jenney: Good.

Anny: You never thought that within – how long have you been here in that chair, let us see okay, about half an hour now, that things could change so fast, huh? You thought it was not possible, don't you? Umm humm.

Stare at my fingers and listen to my voice. Keep your gaze on my fingers and listen to my voice. Your eyelids are getting so heavy, sooooo heavy.

Take a slow deep breath and as you exhalable, close your eyes. And let all your cares fade away, fade away, fade away, fade away, as I am asking for your protection and your well being and I say God, please allow only good thigs to come to Jenney, and for this blessing we give thanks, and now you ask to be placed into the protection of your very own light. Your very own light, your spark of life. It is like a mini sun in your chest. Some people can see it. Some people can feel it. Some people simply know it is there. That light of yours.

That very beautiful light of yours. Let it shine. Let it shine. Let it shine throughout every cell of your body. Throughout your aura. Cleansing your body. Cleansing your aura. Strengthening your body. Strengthening your aura. Extending itself at one arm's length above you, beneath you, at each side of you, in front of you and behind you and mentally repeat with me. This is my body. This is my space. Only light can come to me. Only light can come from me. Only my light can be here.

And as you take a slow deep breath and exhale, go into your head there with your mind. Connect with the pain. Connect with the parts of you who are not feeling good in your head. Connect with them. And in your mind from the bottom of your heart, talk to the cells. Talk to the cells that were shaken up. See them relaxing, relaxing. See them relaxing. In your mind, the work is appropriate for the cells right there to relax. Relax. Relax. Give it some lotion, whatever.

And look at the colour as they are not feeling good. What colour are those cells right there in the head? The cells that are so unhappy. What are the colours of it? What is the colour of it? And I would like to know.

Jenney: Blue.

Anny: It is blue and it is hurting?

Jenney: Yah.

Anny: Have a look at that and in your mind, give it the colour that would relax it. Whatever is the colour that is appropriate. Give it the colour that would relax it. Relax it. And makes it feel fine. And then you will notice what is the temperature that will make them feel really relaxed. And do it too. Do whatever is appropriate so that it feels fine. It feels fine. That is right and to your surprise and delight, the more you make peace with it all, the better it feels in your body and the better it feels inside.

The more you know that things inside are healing beautifully, just like the outside. That is right, just like the outside. And it feels so relaxed, so comfortable, so relaxed, so comfortable. That is right.

The Care Package

And now, you are going to send a care package to the driver of that car. And have a box in front of you. When it is there, let me know. Now put in there how you feel because he ran that red light. Just put it in there. I do not want to hear a thing, it is all in total privacy and give it to him. Huhh. Just put in there how you feel about the whole thing and when you are finished, let me know. (Client was clenching her fists….)

Jenney: (clearing throat). Umm humm.

Anny: All right. Put a picture of you, the way you were when you looked into the mirror at the hospital. Put the picture of you, the way you were and put a picture of you now and (music) each time when you have finished, just let me know.

Jenney: Umm humm.

Anny: Explain to him whatever you want to explain to him about traffic lights, traffic laws and the whole thing.

Jenney: Umm humm.

Anny: Tell him whatever you want to tell him about his way of driving.

Jenney: Umm humm.

Anny: Explain to him how you want him to drive from now on, having a little more respect, uhh huhh, for other people on the road. So tell him how you want him to drive from now on.

Jenney: Umm humm.

Anny: And tell him how you want him to think of you from now on too, and your Mother and the car you were in.

Jenney: Umm humm.

Anny: Now, explain to him something about responsibility as a human being and whatever else you want to tell him.

Jenney: Umm humm.

Anny: And now, just anything else you want to put in there? Because you are going to close the box.

Jenney: Umm humm.

Anny: Explain to him you will be a doctor. And then close the box. (pause) And then you put a label on it from Jenney and when you are ready, let me know.

Jenney: Umm humm.

Anny: Decide how youare going to have that box delivered to him.

Jenney: Umm humm.

Anny: And when it is gone, open your eyes.

Jenney: (eyes open)

Anny: How do you feel now?

Jenney: Relieved.

Anny: You. .

Jenney: My headache is gone.

Anny: You sound surprised. This is a magic chair, huh.

Jenney: Got to be. It is very warm too. My headache has not been gone in one month and it is gone.

Anny: And it is gone. You like it that way?

Jenney: Yah.

Anny: Go into your head and explain to it how much you like it when it feels good like that. And thank it. And totally, totally. Explain to it, it is so nice when it is comfortable. That is right and as you take a slow deep breath and exhale, see yourself graduating from High School. Feeling great. Relax. Getting ready for med school. Just relax. Just relax. That is right. And remember how you felt three months ago. That is right.

And as you take a slow deep breath and exhale, the way you felt three months ago, just transported to now, to tomorrow, that is right. And become aware of your light again.
That light of yours, that mini sun in your chest. That spark of life that you have within you. And explain to that light that you learned a lot. You learned a lot about being a human being and thank it for being there for you. And as you take a slow deep breath and exhale, become more and more relaxed. More and more at peace. More and more relaxed. More and more at peace. Looking forward to the future and enjoying the present. That is right.

Looking forward to the future and truly enjoying the present. Feeling great in every way. And when you are ready, only then will you open your eyes, feeling refreshed, relaxed, renewed, totally at peace with yourself. Totally, totally at peace with yourself and with the world around you. Having learned a great deal. Looking forward to the future. Enjoying the present. Feeling great. Feeling great. And quite surprised. Can you see yourself in med school?

Jenney: Yah.

Anny: Yah. You can see yourself in med school now. That light, trust it. Trust it totally. That is it for today.

Jenney: (Big breath) You know, when I see myself in that car now, I see a white light around me.

Anny: Excellent. Uhh huhh.

Jenney: It is like I am looking at myself and I can see a white light.

Anny: Umm humm. And how does that feel?

Jenney: Safe.

Anny: Yup.

Questions About Zoeh's Session

- Question 1 -
- Question 2 -
- Question 3 -
- Question 4 -
- Question 5 -

Transcript – Zoeh – Warts

First session: 1 hour, including the interview with the Mother.

Zoeh was 7 years old when her doctor sent them to me. She had warts all over both sides of her hands, up to her elbows. The Doctor and the Mother tried everything, including "duct tape", and nothing worked. The condition got worst.

I first interviewed the Mother, alone with me. She explained that at 5 days old, Zoeh had heart surgery. She had lots of allergies, food allergies. Zoeh was very moody and also suffered from eczema.

Zoeh's 9 year old brother was suffering from asthma, eczema and had learning disabilities.

When asked about Zoeh's Grandparents, the Mother explained Zoeh's maternal grandmother died 5 years prior to Zoeh's birth.

Zoeh was wearing long sleeves and very nice lace black gloves, open fingers, long cuffs, Can Can style…

Asking permission to anchor feelings by touching her knees.

Anny: Now Zoeh, I will explain you something. When I will talk. No, and when you will talk, I will touch your knees. It will be a firm touch like that. Sometimes I will touch this knee, sometimes the other, sometimes both and I would like to have your permission to do that? Do you give me permission to touch your knees?

Zoeh: Yah.

Anny: Thank you. You look surprised that I asked that.

Zoeh: No.

Anny: Humm. Your knees. Now can I see your hands. You are hiding them, what is happening with them? Oh, okay, I am getting the idea. Can you lift your – okay

(I wanted to see both sides of her hands and her arms) so that I know. How does it **feel** to have that?

Zoeh: It does not **feel** like anything.

Anny: It does not **feel** like anything? So how come you hide them?

Zoeh: Cause _________ just long sleeve does it.

Anny: Would you like to show your hands?

Zoeh: Yah

Anny: Humm?

Zoeh: Yah.

Anny: You like to show your hands. What is nice about having hands like that?

Zoeh: Umm.

Anny: Humm, what is nice about hands like that if you like to show them?

Zoeh: I do not know.

Anny: Well then you find it nice and you do not know, how come?

Zoeh: Because I do not find it nice.

Anny: You do not find it nice. All right, can you turn your hands. Okay, there are some there too huh?

Zoeh: Umm humm.

Anny: Humm. Okay, let me have a look here. Humm, I am looking here. I would like to see your hand here. How do you **feel** about all this?

Zoeh: Bad.

Anny: Humm?

Zoeh: Bad.

Anny: Okay, now do you know your reason to be here today?

Zoeh: Umm.

Anny: Just to get them away. So that … … did you know that you come here just so that they are gone?

Zoeh: Umm humm.

Anny: And can you explain to me what, what was all the things that were done so that those things are gone. What did you do? What did the doctor do? Your Mom do? What did you do?

Zoeh: My Mom put.

Anny: Humm.

Zoeh: My Mom put garlic on my fork.

Anny: Garlic, okay.

Zoeh: No, garlic and bananas.

Anny: What?
(Client was speaking VERY softly)

Zoeh: Bananas.

Anny: Okay. What did the doctor put on that?

Zoeh: He put like this kind of cream on it.

Anny: And what happened? You do all things like that and what happened?

Zoeh: Nothing.

Anny: Nothing.
(Repeating client to stay out of " it")

Zoeh: It just turned red.

Anny: They just turned red. And how do you **feel** about that?
(Notice: keeping client in her feelings to keep her in a trance)

Zoeh: It **feels** like they were not gone.

(The warts were the focus. Remember: what you focus on is what you get)

Anny: Okay. Zoeh, by the way, my name is Anny. You can call me Anny because that is my name. Okay Zoeh, do you realize something, is that when everybody puts something in there, they are waiting for the stuff that was put there to remove it and it does not work because guess what, you will remove them. <u>Nobody asked you</u> to remove them, yah. Did they? And you know how you are going to remove it?

Zoeh: No.

Anny: With your mind and I am going to help you to do that. Think about it. All the stuff they put there and asking the stuff to remove it. The stuff does not have any brains, so it cannot remove it. And it is like that with eczema and everything. You know you ask something to remove it and it will not. But when you ask your mind to remove it, it will. How do you **feel** about that?

Zoeh: Umm, I do not know.

Anny: Never thought about that? How do you **feel** when you realize that it is your mind that is going to make them go away for good? How do you **feel** about that?

Zoeh: Good.

Anny: Do you think you will **feel** very powerful.

Zoeh: Umm humm.

Anny: Umm humm. Yah. Tell me about school. You go to school?

Zoeh: Umm humm.

Anny: Now, Zoeh, I do not have any children, so I am going to ask you things that you think I should know, but I do not because I do no have any children, so what grade are you?

Zoeh: Grade two.

Anny: Grade two. Grade two at seven years old. Okay, so you started grade one at six, six years old. Okay. What do you like the most about school?

Zoeh: Umm, when I have gym.

Anny: Humm?

Zoeh: When I have gym.

Anny: You like gym. Tell me about that, what is nice about gym?

Zoeh: We play games.

Anny: Humm?

Zoeh: We play games.

Anny: You play games. Umm humm. Very good and anything else you like about school?

Zoeh: Umm, recess...

Anny: Humm?

Zoeh: Recess. I like recess too.

Anny: You like recess too. Very good. And what is it you hate about school? You know I was a little kid one time too and there were things I really liked and things that ohhh. So which one do you hate the most?

Zoeh: Math.

Anny: Math. Okay. What is it about math that you do not like math?

Zoeh: It is hard.

Anny: What? You know I find it interesting because when I was a little girl, math, I loved it. It was like math was talking to me, the numbers, but I was not good at gym. It takes all kinds huh? Anybody at school … … how do you **feel** about your teacher?

Zoeh: She is very nice.

Anny: She is very nice. What makes it that you say so?

Zoeh: Umm.

Anny: I would like you to speak a little louder so that I do not have to bend like that. What is nice about your teacher?

Zoeh: When somebody in our class gets hurt

Anny: Yes.

Zoeh: She cares a lot about them.

Anny: She cares. That's nice huh.

Zoeh: Umm humm.

Anny: Who do you care for the most?

Zoeh: My best friend, Shirley.

Anny: Your best friend Shirley, tell me about Shirley.

Zoeh: Umm.

Anny: What is about her that you like her? She is your best friend. What makes her your best friend?

Zoeh: She always shares.

Anny: Is that right. Now, I understand that you have a brother. What is his first name?

Zoeh: Whose first name?

Anny: Humm?

Zoeh: Whose first name?

Anny: Your brother's first name. How do you call your brother? You have a brother do you not? you? Do you? What is his name? What is your brother's name?

Zoeh: Bodies?

Anny: I did not understand that. What is it?

Zoeh: Did you say bodies?

Anny: Your brother. You have a brother?

Zoeh: Umm humm.

Anny: What is his name?

Zoeh: Rowley.

Anny: Rowley?

Zoeh: Yah, Rowley.

Anny: Do you know how you spell that?

Zoeh: R O W L E Y.

Anny: V Y.

Zoeh: L E Y.

Anny: ROW. And the first name is? "V" like Victor or "R" like Robert?

Zoeh: His first name is Rowley.

Anny: No the first letter of his name?

Zoeh: R.

Anny: R, like Robert?

Zoeh: Umm humm.

Anny: Or Robin. Rowley, that is it?

Zoeh: Umm humm.

Anny: Okay, very good. What do you **feel** about him?

Zoeh: Umm, he is umm, he is nice.

Anny: Humm.

Zoeh: He is nice.

Anny: Is he nice to you?

Zoeh: Umm humm.

Anny: Okay, tell me what he does that he is nice to you.

Zoeh: Umm. At Halloween, he shares candy with me.

Anny: What?

Zoeh: At Halloween, he shares candy with me.

Anny: Okay, so now, are you ready? Now I'm going to ask you something. Maybe for you. … … you would like, you do what you want, okay: Maybe it will be better for you to close your eyes and talk to your hands. Which one would like to be, like to have a nice smooth hand – which one of the two?

Zoeh: This one.

Anny: That one. Okay.
Okay, today left hand and also all the way – can you lift your thing and I would like to see both sides there? So all the way to the elbow, okay.
So make sure, well you know, left hand, left arm, so it does not matter where it stops. Okay. And left arm.

It is your mind who is going to do it. That is how come all the things they put there did not work. Because everybody thinks that something else is going to do it for us, and you know, life is not like that.
Okay, very good. What game do you like to play the most?

Zoeh: Humm, Clue.

Anny: Can you explain me how you play that game.

Zoeh: First you can be Mrs. Peacock or Mr. Plumb or umm, Mrs. White and some other players and umm, you roll the dice and whoever gets the biggest number goes first. And then let us say you pick six and I mean there is different ones, but if you pick six and you get into the room, you can see that umm, Rowley do you got Mrs. Peacock with a knife in the whatever room you are in and then you have to guess what is in the envelope.

Anny: Umm humm. Are you good at it?

Zoeh: Umm humm.

Anny: How does that **feel** to be good at it?

Zoeh: Good because it is only for ten and up, but I can still play it.

Anny: Is that right. Okay, so now – do you have a computer at home?

Zoeh: Umm humm.

Anny: Do you know when there is something on the screen how to delete it, you know.

Zoeh: Umm humm.

Anny: To make it go away.

Zoeh: At school we have that kind of computer that if you are in something you can go delete it, but in our computer I di not try it because you have to go into the internet to do it.

Anny: Okay, very good. Now, you, as I explain to you, I am going to help you with it so I am going to ask you to just, you know how your hand and your arm looks like, do you not?

Zoeh: Umm humm.

Anny: So it is okay, you can put that back like that so it is more comfortable for you. Okay, so now, umm humm. By the way, do you trust me?

Zoeh: Umm humm.

Anny: Thank you. All right.

Okay let me because I want to understand how you think so that I can help you with this. I am asking your mind to do something here. All right. In your mind find yourself in front of the computer and on the computer is your left hand – your left. Can you see it in your mind? Tell me when you know, you know it is like somebody took a picture and you put your hand like that in front, inside of the computer and you can see it. Can you do that? Because you are going to play with the computer and every wart on your hand you can see it and you know the computer they can move things and you can see it. And you know playing and deleting all of them, one after the other and only on this arm and this hand. So, can you do that? You can close your eyes if you like it, or if you do not want to, you do not have to, it is up to you.
And tell me how is it for you to see yourself deleting, deleting, deleting. Do you know what I am talking about. Can you do that?

Zoeh: Umm humm.

Anny: You tell me if you can. If you cannot, tell me too. Can you see yourself deleting you know?

Zoeh: Umm humm.

Anny: All those round things there you know. There you are, delete, delete, delete, delete. All the way until your skin is nice and smooth, nice and smooth. In your mind, so maybe it is easier for you to not have your eyes open for that. Maybe it will be easier to have your eyes closed, I do not know because it depends the people. Some people it is easier with your eyes open. Some people it is easier with your eyes closed. Can you see yourself deleting? I am going to put some music on so that each time you delete, there is a sound. You know because computers do that, huh?

Zoeh: Umm humm.

Anny: They have sound. I am going to, just a moment, to put a sound here. (Crystal Cavern music on) You see and each crystal sound is one of those round things there disappearing, disappearing. In your mind. You do that in your mind. Click, it makes a crystal sound and it is disappears. It is almost like a bubble that just burst and it feels so good. It feels so good. And with the pointer, you point on one and you make delete and it makes a sound, just like a bubble that bursts. And you become so relaxed, so relaxed, so relaxed, so relaxed. So relaxed that as you are doing that, are you doing it?

Zoeh: Umm humm.

Anny: And how does it **feel** to be able to delete it like that? How does it **feel?** And when you are finished with one side of the hand, you turn it on the other side. Turn it over and you delete and you say, there is one there. Delete. One there. You see and then there is one there. And then in your mind you see them just going. It is going and it **feels** so good. It **feels** so good and in your mind, **feel** your skin becoming smoother and smoother and smoother and smoother. In your mind and you can **feel**, really **feel**, your skin becoming nice and smooth. Nice and smooth, nice and smooth, nice and smooth. And when in your mind your hand and your arm, the skin of your hands and your arm are smooth, you tell me when you deleted them all, let me know. In your mind see a nice smooth skin. How is it going?

You have to tell me because it is your mind, so I do not know when you have it done – finished.

Zoeh: I am finished now.

Anny: Finished now. How was it for you to look at that. Delete, and it is gone. How is that for you? You have to tell me because I want to make sure that I gave you all the ideas so that your mind is doing it.

Zoeh: It **feels** good.

Anny: It **feels** what?

Zoeh: It **feels** good.

Anny: It **feels** good. How does it **feel**? How does **feel** good **feels**? Tell me. How does that **feel**, **feeling** good? Because you see, you **feeling** good is one **feeling**. For me **feeling** good is another **feeling**. If it is **feeling** good. I have my way of **feeling** good. You have your way of **feeling** good. So I would like to know how do you **feel?** How does it **feel** to **feel** good?

Zoeh: Nice.

Anny: Umm humm. You like that?

Zoeh: Umm humm.

Anny: ***(Wrapping it up, sealing it in, so to speak)*** Can you breathe in the nice **feeling**. Breathe it in, breathe it in and breathe it into your hand and your arm. Just breathe in the good **feeling** in your hand and in your arm.

Just breathe it in, just breathe it in and enjoy it. And breathe the good **feeling** and **feeling** of a nice smooth skin. A very nice and smooth skin and then you can go call your Mom because I am going to talk to your Mom to give her some ideas to make life easier to all of you. Would you like that?

Zoeh: Yah.

Anny: Humm?

Zoeh: Umm humm.

Anny: But I am going to first stop the recoding and give it to you because it is yours.

Zoeh: Okay.

Anny: All right. Watch your feet, here and you can get off the chair okay.

(Remember, at that point, client perceives the session is over and have their guards down, thus very open to suggestions.)

Almost ready to leave the consultation room, I asked client if she was taking a bath or a shower. Surprised, she said she takes a bath.

Then, I said with lots of gestures " Zoeh, from now on each time the plug is removed to let the water drain, it will take down the drain everything that has to be removed, cleansing your body, so your skin is nice and smooth from the top of your head to the tip of your toes."

Once alone with client's mother, we wrote a script together, a "sleep therapy" script, asking the mother to read it to her daughter when she was 15 minutes into her sleep.

The script was about feeling comfortable, breathing easily, enjoying being alive.

It was important to have the mother re-enforce the suggestions given to Client. The solution is to give a “prescription”. I asked the mother to make a very strong decaffeinated herbal tea of a colour that will impress Zoeh’s mind. 4 to 5 bags for a cup of tea. It must have a strong taste. Making sure she is alone when she does this, pour the tea in a bottle with an eyedropper, and give 2 drops of that concoction on Zoeh’s tongue before going to bed, repeating what I had written on a label to be glued to the bottle:

TO HAVE A NICE SMOOTH SKIN.

And in the morning, ask Zoeh to drink a glass of water to flush out whatever has to be flushed out so that she has a NICE SMOOTH SKIN.

Please note this is important because the mother was only talking about WARTS, and I wanted to only talk about a smooth skin or not having a smooth skin. ***(The warts were the focus. Remember: what you focus on is what you get. It was important to shift the focus on a smooth skin.)***

At the second visit about two weeks later, this time to deal with the asthma, Zoeh had a nice smooth skin. Although my suggestions were for only one arm (The idea was one limb at the time so Zoeh could adjust comfortably to the new look), almost all the warts on her body were gone.

Her mother explained that after taking a bath, the bottom of the bathtub was covered with warts as she pulled the plug to let the water drain and that Zoeh would stand in the bathtub and scream at the sight, with her mother reassuring her that the water was taking down the drain everything that has to be removed, cleansing her body, so that she has a skin nice and smooth from the top of her head to the tip of her toes. ***And it did.***

Questions About Ethan's Session

- Question 1 -
- Question 2 -
- Question 3 -
- Question 4 -
- Question 5 -

Transcript – Ethan (7 Years Old) Attitude And Food

Anny: Like this. Yup. This is all right. Now Erhan.

Ethan: Yah.

Anny: I learned a lot of things to do through the years and I learned what is the best thing. Leave that alone, okay. I learned what makes things much easier. So when I do this type of work. So, one of the things I do is touch the knees. It is to be a firm touch like that. Some times I will touch this knee, some times the other and some times both and I would like to have your permission to do that.

Ethan: Of course.

Anny: Well thank you. They are your knees.

Ethan: I know but.

Anny: Yah, well I am asking permission. So.

Ethan: I already gave the answer.

Anny: Well we have to wait till that plane is past so we can hear ourselves.

Ethan: I can hear you perfectly.

Anny: Very good and you do not have to, the mike picks up pretty good. Now I would like to tell me something. What is that fancy thing about vegetables?

Ethan: Well, I do not really like that many vegetables. But I do like peas and stuff, but.

Anny: You like peas.

Ethan: Carrots. Yah, like you know those little green peas.

Anny: Yes.

Ethan: But I do not like carrots, broccoli. Like green and orange vegetables. The only..

Anny: You do not like. Do not like green and orange vegetables.

Ethan: Except for peas.

Anny: Oh yes, except for peas. Okay, I am going to say peas are very good, I understand that because you know.

Ethan: Peas do have a good taste.

Anny: They have a very good taste, yup.

Ethan: Especially when they are still in those pea pod things.

Anny: Yes, it is really good then, yuh. Okay now, so, but there are some vegetables that are, for example, there are green, purple, there are yellow. How are you with that? Do you eat them?

Ethan: Ah, ah, I was, I never knew green vegetables, I mean yellow vegetables ever existed.

Anny: Yes, there are. And mushrooms, they are almost white.

Ethan: Oh yah, mushrooms, but.

Anny: Talk about mushrooms.

Ethan: Well you know, well I do not have a very good taste for things that grow out of the ground that much.

Anny: That grow what?

Ethan: Out of the ground. You know how mushrooms grow out of the grounds. Peas do, but I do have a good taste for them, but mushrooms, kind of well …

Anny: What things?

Ethan: Well mushrooms kind of just…

Anny: What is it about it?

Ethan: I do not know, I just do not know.

Anny: Oh yes you do, otherwise. Do not tell me you do something you do not know. Huh huh.

Ethan: Well…

Anny: Listen, I will tell you something. I learned by doing this that boys and girls of your age are very smart.

Ethan: That is true.

Anny: The thing is that it is quite interesting what they are using it for.

Ethan: Hum.

Anny: What game are you playing?

Ethan: What do you mean, what game?

Anny: Yah, you are playing a game.

Ethan: Oh no I am not (laughing).

Anny: Oh yes. You are playing a game at making a scene of I do not know. You are playing a game.

Ethan: (laughing) I am not playing a game.

Anny: Yes you do.

Ethan: (laughing)

Anny: So, because if you did not, you would eat a little bit. Because then you would learn something.

Ethan: Well about mushrooms, well, they just kind of taste funny. That I really do not like things that taste funny to me.

Anny: Well everything tastes funny.

Ethan: No, not everything.

Anny: Oh sure.

Ethan: Not hotdogs. Not smokies. Not macaroni and cheese. They do not, those things do not taste funny. And some other things don't taste funny to me. It's just…

Anny: Okay what is it about it that taste funny. You tell me.

Ethan: Well, it is mostly the colors because I can….

Anny: Well you told me that and you just told me that it is just something, from what you explained to me. You told me it is just an excuse.

Ethan: No, I did not.

Anny: Yah, because first you say you do not like green or orange vegetables. Well, there are red peppers. They are bright red. Do you like them? There are purples that are beautiful yellow. Do you like them? Mushrooms, they are almost white. Do you like them? So do not give me that.

Ethan: Well, actually I do not like mushrooms.

Anny: Because?

Ethan: Just because. That is the answer I give you.

Anny: That is the truth, just because. Okay. Now would you like to know really what it is about that you do not like instead of what you say.

Ethan: Actually, actually what I say is true cause how do you know?

Anny: Well, would you like to find out?

Ethan: Sure.

Anny: Are you sure. You might have a good laugh you know.

Ethan: (laughing) I am sure.

Anny: You are sure. All right, but something else I would like to know. Okay how come you are brought here because you do not like vegetables. Well you can, there is one thing, you cannot like vegetables but eat them just a little bit any way.

Ethan: Yah (laughing) I can not.

Anny: Will you do that?

Ethan: Yah.

Anny: You do?

Ethan: Most of the time, but some times it takes me quite a while.

Anny: Yah.

Ethan: Most of the time it takes me until after dessert, which is a long time after dinner. So some times it even takes me after dessert, which is a long time in my house. Takes a while.

Anny: And what happen when you do not eat vegetables. First of all where are you when you are asked to eat vegetables?

Ethan: I am usually at the kitchen table and when I do not eat my vegetables, I am asked to go to my room and sit in my bed quite a while, which gets pretty annoying, and it drives me crazy.

Anny: So what is so nice about being sent to your room and make you absolutely crazy?

Ethan: That I have to sit on my bed for a while, which makes me very crazy.

Anny: Yah, the thing is what is nice about it?

Ethan: What is nice about it? Nothing is nice about it.

Anny: Oh yes, because if it was not nice, you would eat the vegetables instead of going into your room.

Ethan: Well some times I just choose to do that.

Anny: Ethan, what is nice about being sent to your room?

Ethan: That I get…

Anny: Who sends you to your room?

Ethan: My Dad. Either my Dad, my Mother or my Grandma.

Anny: Your grandma also. So what is nice about being sent to your room?

Ethan: Well, I get a nice feel when I look out the window.

Anny: You see. I told you that I do that for a long time.

Ethan: (laughing).

Anny: And I told you we are going to have a good laugh.

Ethan: (laughing)

Anny: So you want to go to look at the window and everything huh?

Ethan: Yah.

Anny: So you want to go to your room.

Ethan: Yah, but not all the time I want to go.

Anny: And so when you do not want to go, what happens?

Ethan: I just take a while to eat my vegetables and I do it. But peas of course would only take me four or five. It would take me only six or seven minutes. But carrots and broccoli, probably four hours.

Anny: Umh.

Ethan: Either three or four hours. Maybe half an hour.

Anny: Okay, so would you like to know. You see. Um hum.

Ethan: Would I like to know what?

Anny: All right. What I would like you to do Ethan is in your mind see yourself at the table, at the kitchen table in your home. And in your mind here you are at the table and you are told, well you are given vegetables.

Ethan: What type?

Anny: I do not know. You choose the one.

Ethan: I choose peas.

Anny: Okay, you choose peas. And as peas are given to you, I would like you to check inside of your body. How does it feel inside?

Ethan: Well the peas taste pretty good.

Anny: Yah, well how does it feel inside when you see peas?

Ethan: Well, I feel normal. Normal actually. Can I open my eyes now?

Anny: You can open your eyes. I never asked you to close them.

Ethan: Oh. You want me to think about a different vegetables?

Anny: First of all the peas. You chose the peas, we are going to stick with the peas. How does it feel inside?

Ethan: I already told you my answer. Normal.

Anny: I did not get it. Normal. And how does it feel to feel normal?

Ethan: Well, my tummy kind of like aches and stuff. Which is normal.

Anny: You what?

Ethan: My tummy kind of aches just this much, which is normal. But usually it aches this much.

Anny: Ummmm.

Ethan: But my tummy aches this much. And when I eat my tummy aches this much and well, I guess I just feel like ..

Anny: Okay, now all right. Imagine here are broccolis and how does it feel inside?

Ethan: It feels like I am going to blow up. And that is also about carrots.

Anny: How do you feel the blow up?

Ethan: Actually….

Anny: Put your hand on it.

Ethan: When I blow up. Can I imagine so that I can feel more about that.

Anny: Hum?

Ethan: Can I just imagine so I can feel more about that?

Anny: Sure. Yup. Just imagine so you can feel more about it.

Ethan: Well, when I feel like I am going to blow up, I feel so. I feel like a volcano, which is so hard. Well I just automatically just stop. I feel like I am going to blow up in two seconds.

Anny: Okay, thank you. Well now. We are going to put your hands like this on your lap and make it comfortable, okay, like this. So that you are comfortable and by the way. I am going to ask you to sit a little differently because like that you are sitting on your spine and that is not good. Here like this. Okay. Now.

Ethan: When you kind of moved me, you kind of hurt this part of me. That always happens when I get picked up from there. Like not like this high, but even when I am just being moved a little, it hurts, when someone picks me from there.

Anny: Okay, well next time I will pick you up a different way, okay. So now, in one hand, you are going to put the part that feels normal. That when you are at the table and something is given to you.

Ethan: Well, it is…

Anny: I would like you to choose one hand. The part of you who feels normal when the tummy….

Ethan: It is always my back. Like.

Anny: That feels normal?

Ethan: It is always my back.

Anny: When you are given peas when you are at the table and you told me that you have peas for example, it feels normal inside, right. Put it in one hand. You choose the hand.

Ethan: I am choosing this hand and

Anny: Okay.

Ethan: Can I just do this for all my body.

Anny: Yup, it is fine. Okay you hold it like this because we are going to talk to it. And in the other hand I would like you to put the part of you that feels like volcano, ready to blow up in seconds and put your hands like this - you are holding it. So here you are holding the part of you who feels normal.

Ethan: Ummm.

Anny: Umm, well then change hands. So that is the part of you who feels normal and that is the part of you who feels ready to blow up?

Ethan: Well it is kind of me cut in half. You know how some times it is okay on the palm and okay on the top.

Anny: So it is part of your root and it feels cut in half, okay.

Ethan: Yah.

Anny: Well, so the part. Which is the part that is ready to blow up?

Ethan: Up here.

Anny: Okay, well then you are holding your hand like this and that here, you are hold your hand like this, but you know you can hold it just like that. Because it is important that you feel comfortable. So it is almost ….

Ethan: I do feel comfortable up here.

Anny: Okay, so all right. Humm.

Ethan: And this is where the cutting in half begins.

Anny: Is not that interesting. All right. So I am going to ask the part that is ready to blow up. What is nice and that part is going to explain to that part here who feels good. What is nice about being ready to blow up?

Ethan: Well pretty much that I will not have to eat my vegetables for the rest of my life. Especially broccoli.

Anny: Can you tell me that again, because I find that very interesting. Okay leave that alone here. That part and you talk to me. Well you are going to talk to that part. That part here who is ready to blow up is going to talk to that part what? Repeat it again.

Ethan: Well, when. Could you ask the question like before you asked me if.

Anny: Well if you would listen, you will get it. Tell the part I am going to ask the part that is ready to blow up because it has to eat broccoli, the carrots and things like that, to tell the part here that feels good, normal, what is nice about being ready to blow up?

Ethan: Well, that once I blow up I will never have to eat my vegetables again.

Anny: And.

Ethan: And that is about it.

Anny: I do not think so, because you said something else before.

Ethan: That is what I said before.

Anny: No. You said something about having to eat your vegetables for the rest of your life.

Ethan: Oh, that is if I do not blow up, I will have to eat vegetables. Well actually it is really not what I like, except for peas of course. Ummm. Huh.

Anny: You are quite a game player are you no i?

Ethan: Well some times.

Anny: So, what is it about it that you think if you eat it now, you will have to eat it for the rest of your life. Where does that idea come from?

Ethan: Well pretty much not the rest of my life, like that's not all I am going to eat, but when Dad is home, yup. I am going to have to eat a lot. Only for two weeks anyways.

Anny: What do you mean for two weeks?

Ethan: Dad is down north for two weeks and Dad is home for weeks.

Anny: And what happens when he is gone?

Ethan: Well, I do not have to eat as many vegetables. I can have more meat.
Anny: So, and when he is there?

Ethan: Well, we get the same amount of vegetables. Well almost because vegetables gets a little higher than meat.

Anny: Is that right?

Ethan: But…

Anny: In your mind?

Ethan: When Dad is gone, vegetables gets down really low and meat gets really high.

Anny: All right you told me that you do not eat them, so do not tell me you are eating them anyway.

Ethan: That, well I said..

Anny: Listen, just keep. I have had enough of this. Okay. I want you to tell me the truth.

Ethan: Some times I don't feel like it.

Anny: Okay, what for? What makes it that makes you do not feel like it?

Ethan: Well pretty much some, well pretty much it is a secret and I do not really tell my secrets.

Anny: Repeat that again.

Ethan: Pretty much they are secrets and I do not tell my secrets to anyone.

Anny: What is the secret you are not telling anyone?

Ethan: Well if I told you, it would not be a secret would it?

Anny: I told you that the only person it is going to say it is me. I want to understand you. I find it very interesting. So the real reason is a secret, huh. Umm hummm. So you know the reason you do it, do you not? And what are the results. What happen when you are doing it?

Ethan: Could you repeat that again, I did not quite catch it all.

Anny: What happen when you do it and you get your way?

Ethan: Well pretty much I feel happy, but when I do not get my way, I feel a little bit happy and little bit sad and mad, all at the same time.

Anny: So it is your way, or no way?

Ethan: No, it is my way or Mommy and Daddy's way and when it is Mommy and Daddy's way, I do not like the way it is. I get a little mad, which makes me go to my room and not let anyone in for quite awhile.

Anny: Okay and how old is Ethan? Deep inside, who is that way?

Ethan: Repeat that, I did not quite…

Anny: Inside of you, how old is Ethan who feels that way.

Ethan: My age, seven years old.

Anny: I do not think so, because you start that earlier than that. So you are a seven year old acting like what, a baby who likes to have it his way or no way?

Ethan: A four year old actually.

Anny: A four year old, okay.

Ethan: Cause that is when it all began.

Anny: That is when what began? It all began when you were four?

Ethan: Yes, and I ca not remember that far back, but

Anny: Oh yes you do.

Ethan: I remember some of that far back.

Anny: Can you tell me some of it?

Ethan: Well I remember I was going to daycare and stuff. Which is almost all I could remember.

Anny: Okay, tell me about it.

Ethan: Daycare?

Anny: Umh hum. Daycare, tell me about daycare. Because you see, I am not from this country. I have no idea what is daycare.

Ethan: Daycare is like after school when you have, when your parents have to go somewhere and you ca not stay home cause there is no one to look after, you go to daycare.

Anny: Okay I did not know that. Okay and then what happened in daycare?

Ethan: Well, there is a whole bunch of things up there. There is staff, there is snack time, there is lunch and there is also a lot of playing and you get to go the park and you get field trips and stuff and you get some visitors from different places, like Christie the Clown whose running away from the circus.

Anny: How did you like that?

Ethan: Well it was pretty fun, actually.

Anny: I must say, but what does that have to do with vegetables. It is not vegetables really. It is making you do something that you do not want to do.

Ethan: (laughing) Well.

Anny: What does that have to do with that?

Ethan: Well daycare has to do somethings with that because sometimes during snack time there is vegetables, especially carrots.

Anny: Especially carrots.

Ethan: I mean like there is also carrots.

Anny: Yes, oh yah, oh yah, oh yah. Is not that interesting. Tell me more about all that. Remember I do not know a thing about it. I do not have any kids and I am not from this country. So I am very surprised about that.

Ethan: Do not you have daycares in Africa?

Anny: No.

Ethan: Not even anything that.

Anny: Oh yes, I went to school over there, but it was kindergarten. You go to kindergarten from age three, which I went to school since I am three years old, but there was no daycare.

Ethan: You mean you always had to stay home?

Anny: Yup. My Mom and Dad would take me all kinds of places though.

Ethan: Even in business places?

Anny: Yes, because my Dad was in business.

Ethan: Oh interesting.

Anny: So, anyway, tell me more about daycare. What is it about daycare that you did not like?

Ethan: That you get in trouble quite a bit.

Anny: You do what quite a bit?

Ethan: Some times you get into trouble quite a bit. Like some times even the whole day you get into trouble.

Anny: What was nice about that?

Ethan: Nothing really.

Anny: Yes, otherwise you would not get into trouble.

Ethan: Hey I am new to this. Take your daycare, I do not know all the rules.

Anny: And so what happens when you know all the rules?

Ethan: Well as Courtland, he is the one that is been to daycare the longest of all the daycare. He knows all the rules the best and he does not follow them that much.

Anny: He what?

Ethan: He does follow the rules, but not all the time.

Anny: And what does that have to do with Ethan?

Ethan: I am kind of like Courtland and even though I have never been there the longest, I do kind of act like Courtland.

Anny: Is not that interesting and you just like a sheep heh?

Ethan: Baaaahhhh.

Anny: Yah, he does it, I follow.

Ethan: No, not all the time.

Anny: And then. Well that is what you told me.

Ethan: I said some times.

Anny: And what is the thing he did?

Ethan: Well, he gets into trouble.

Anny: And what is nice about getting into trouble?

Ethan: You should ask Courtland, cause he is the one that chooses.

Anny: But you are the one that does the same.

Ethan: Not all the time.

Anny: But you decided to do the same. What was nice about it?

Ethan: Well, I do not know.

Anny: Yes you do.

Ethan: How do you know?

Anny: I do this for a very long time.

Ethan: (laughing) But some time some people do not even know the answers.

Anny: Yes they do.

Ethan: To explain their own thing.

Anny: Uhh, to explain. They do not know how to explain, but they know the answer.

Ethan: Well right now I do not know how to explain either.

Anny: Okay, well find out a way to explain it to me.

Ethan: I can explain to you that it'is a secret.

Anny: Oh yah. And?

Ethan: And, I do not tell my secrets. Some of them I do, but not all them. And that is one of the secrets I don't tell.

Anny: Umm humm. I figured that.

Ethan: Can we start talking about some fruits now?

Anny: Some what?

Ethan: Some fruits.

Anny: Well tell me about fruit. Your way or no way, huh? You want me to talk about fruit, well go ahead.

Ethan: Hahhh. Well some fruits I like. Just as vegetables, some fruits I like some fruits I do not. Besides talking about vegetables is getting a little boring.

Anny: Yah, you like to entertain yourself do you not?

Ethan: (laughing) Yah.

Anny: That is the big secret huh. It is too smooth, it gets boring. Um?

Ethan: Umh hum.

Anny: Umh hum. I told you I do that for a long time.

Ethan: But you never - you have not heard of daycare for a long time.

Anny: I never heard about daycare. You are the first one who told me about it. Because you are the first one who talked about it. Because usually when people your age come to make life easier for them, they do other things. You are doing that, but the result is all the same. So when I tell them I am going to tell your Mother to just back off, say nothing. They are shocked. They don not like it because then there is no more entertainment.

Ethan: Some entertainment I do not like.

Anny: Hum?

Ethan: Some entertainment I do not like.

Anny: Which one do you not like?

Ethan: Well, pretty much all of it but I like half the amount of entertainment in the world, but the other half.

Anny: Tell me which one you like.

Ethan: Well, I like circus entertainment and when I go to Florida where they do dances and they dress up like Disney stars. Like the Lion King. They do a little show about that. I like that kind of entertainment.

Anny: And what is it that you do not like?

Ethan: Of entertainment? Well, I really d no't like in a different country they do something like sword swallowing, like those people do that with swords. I do not like that kind.

Anny: Okay you do not like it. Now how does it feel at home when everything is nice and smooth?

Ethan: What does smooth mean?

Anny: Smooth is that everybody is happy. You know everything is quiet.

Ethan: That is barely ever. That barely ever happens. Well

Anny: What would happen if it happens?

Ethan: Well, the same thing that you said. Everyone would be happy and everything would be quiet, but usually everybody would fight and get mad.

Anny: And how does that feel?

Ethan: Very bad because some times I do not like when they fight. Like with Charlene. I do not like when people fight with Charlene or when Charlene fights with others. Because I just do not like when people fight. How can these things actually happen if no one is going to know about them?

Anny: Humm?

Ethan: How can these things happen if no one is going to know about them?

Anny: I do not know.

Ethan: They are not going to happen if no one knows about them. So you should tell Mom about…
Anny: I do not tell your Mom anything. I told you that before. That is how come you can say anything on that recording. I know all what you are doing at the moment is telling things you want your Mom to know and you know what?

Ethan: What?

Anny: It will not happen. Because you are not telling me the truth. You are telling me what you want me to tell your Mother. And to tell you the truth, I am not impressed.

Ethan: Why, I like when people tell about things.

Anny: Yes, now because you are not telling me the truth. You are telling me what you want me to tell your Mother and I told you I will not. And I know if you fake it or if you tell me the truth. And I told you, I am not impressed. I see a lot of children here and I can tell you. I can tell the difference. Yup. Umm hummm. So what is so nice about making a fuss about what you even fake something.

Ethan: Sorry I did not catch that.

Anny: What is so nice about making such a scene about everything. Including what you are doing in this chair at the moment. What is so nice about it?

Ethan: That I can keep some of my secrets.

Anny: I could not care less about your secrets to tell you the truth.

Ethan: You do not know of them.

Anny: I know much more than you think.

Ethan: Yah.

Anny: Because a secret is what you do not tell me and I know what you tell me, so I know what you are not telling me. So I know the secret.

Ethan: Yah, but some things you are not asking me about, so you do not know that those things are a secret.

Anny: Well what is it that I should ask you to know if it is a secret or not?

Ethan: Nothing, I do not like. I already told you, I do not like telling my secrets.

Anny: And what would happen if you did tell them?

Ethan: Well, I would go straight to my room and close the door and I would not let anyone in for a couple of minutes.

Anny: I wonder what would happen if your Mom and Dad would not let you in the house for a couple of minutes because they have a secret.

Ethan: Well they would tell me to wait outside and then I would and…

Anny: Which is exactly what I am going to do with your Mom. How does it feel.

Ethan: I do not know.

Anny: A taste of your own medicine huh?

Ethan: What about a taste of your own medicine?

Anny: What?

Ethan: What about a taste of your own medicine?
Anny: What about what?

Ethan: What about a taste of your own medicine?

Anny: No. It is not my stuff. It is your is. So it is your medicine, not mine. And you want your Mom to know that because of what you are saying on this recording and you think she will not know that is something I will tell. I will tell her that you did not say a word of truth because everything you said, you made sure it was on the recording so she would listen to it. Umm humm. I will tell her that and you can go now.

Ethan: Okay.

Anny: Bye. Just a minute put your feet on top here.

Questions About Gil Boyne's Session

- Question 1 -

- Question 2 -

- Question 3 -

- Question 4 -

- Question 5 -

Transcript – Gil Boyne – Using Hypnosis In A Hospital Setting

I am Gil Boyne, and welcome to the newest in our series featuring new and creative applications of hypnosis and hypnotherapy. Our guest today is a certified respiratory therapist. Let us meet him now.

John: Hi Gil.

Gil: John, it is a pleasure having you back. About 7 years ago, you showed up here at the Institute and you wanted to start the training in hypnotism and hypnotherapy.

John: That is right Gil.

Gil: At that time, what was your motive? Many of the people come here to consider a career change. Others are learning to use hypnosis within an existing career. What was your motive and your plans for using hypnosis back there in 1976?

John: Well at the time Gil, I had been in the field for a number of years, respiratory field. And I found that there were times when drugs or conventional therapy were ineffective in giving the patient the comfort and relief that they desired. So I began to research on my own through reading and through association alternative methods to provide these patients with the relief and the comfort that they wanted so much.

Gil: Once you began, or let me say, once you finished your training, some months later, you accumulated 200 hours of professional training in the hypnosis hypnotherapy, did you immediately begin to use it in the hospital and if you did, were you able to use it openly? And, was there any resistance from physicians, nurses or other healthcare professionals? That is a three part question.

John: Well as soon as I was capable of providing the hypnotic induction, I went into the hospital in Santa Monica where I was working and began to hypnotize fellow healthcare professionals. And I did this either in a group situation or on an individual basis.

Gil: So you were getting practice and developing a professional reputation at the same time.

John: Tthat is right. And I found the response was so enthusiastic that I continued to do so. And eventually by word of mouth some of the physicians that were overseeing our department began to become aware of this technique that I was introducing. My next step was to introduce the technique to the physician. In other words, I asked the physician if it was okay for me to hypnotize one of his patients in front of the doctor. I then in turn . . .

Gil: And that is called direct supervision.

John: That is correct. I in turn took the physician into the patient's room and did a hypnotic induction in front of the physician. The physician was quite impressed and from that moment on there was a snowballing effect of progressively more work as far as hypnotic inductions.

Gil: And what happened finally when this knowledge of your use of hypnosis in hospital settings with these patients, what happened when the hospital administrators learned of it?

John: Well there was quite an uproar in the beginning because there was a misunderstanding of what I was doing and why I was doing it. And also there was a misunderstanding or a total lack of understanding of the subject matter, in this case hypnotism. So what I did is I sat down and I wrote a protocol, a direction that we would take as a department in introducing hypnotism to the patients in the hospital. I in turn submitted this protocol to the executive medical committee of the hospital and they reviewed it and found it to be quite appropriate and authorized me to be, to go out and hypnotize patients under physician's approval.

Gil: Now you were working then as I understand it, primarily with asthmatics, post-surgical and people with other respiratory problems, is that correct?

John: That is right, they were either chronically diseased or they had suffered some sort of trauma, either through surgical practice or accident.

Gil: When you developed your protocol, were you then able to begin training others in the hospital setting?

John: Yes after a period of time there was such an interest and a curiosity and a desire to be a part of what I was doing that I began to hold regular classes for other healthcare professionals and in these classes these healthcare professionals were taught reinforcing techniques so that they in turn could reinforce the positive relief-giving post-hypnotic suggestions that I left with the patient.

Gil: From the time that you first introduced it until you had an approved protocol and were teaching other healthcare providers in the hospital setting, what was the time interval? How long did it take you to market hypnosis in the hospital?

John: Well Again, once I learned to hypnotize, make a hypnotic induction, I began immediately. And on a sort of unauthorized scale, I was doing that. In other words, I wasn't given a blanket approval or written approval but it was known to hospital officials that I was providing these services. That went on for about three months. After about three months I submitted a written program that took about two months for approval.

Gil: And in your written program, did you then have reports and evaluations of what had happened with the work you had been doing?

John: Yes I did include documentation as far as patients worked with previously and the results.

Gil: And what happened?

John: A very favourable response. And not only that, the physicians of the patients that I worked with voluntarily submitted written endorsements of my work. And that presented a very strong case to the hospital administrators.

Gil: Well I am delighted to have you back and now we are going to move right into the video portion of your training program utilizing slides that you shot right there in the hospital setting.

John: Yes. I would like to add, Gil, that the slides you are about to see are demonstrations of actual hypnotic inductions in the hospital environments and these techniques have proven to be most effective so I urge your viewers to watch closely.

Gil: Alright let's look now at our training program developed and created by John Silvas who we just met and we call this program the "Creative Use of Hypnosis in a Hospital Setting by Non Physicians."

First, communicate with the requesting physician to make sure he has written an order for your services in the patient chart. This is important to both you and the physician. Once this is done, you will want to familiarize yourself with the patient's physical complaint as well as the planned clinical course the patient will be subjected to. This information can be found in the patient's chart, under the section marked Patient History. Your next step will be to make contact with the patient's nurse. The nurse will be a vital link between you and the patient. For the nurse can provide you with invaluable information regarding the patient's physical and mental status, as well as how you might best be able to help the patient. For example, information about the patient's sleeping habits, or stress responses, or even resistance to your presence. Also, it is extremely important to set up a schedule regarding the time of day that you will be working with the patient, because there are many services provided to the patient throughout the day by different healthcare providers. Once this is done, it is time to enter the patient's room. When you do, it is advisable to take a moment to observe the patient's physical condition from a short distance, so that you can assess the patient's physical state of comfort or discomfort without influencing their behaviour.

From this distance, you can observe any potential signs of stress or distress or even anxiety. Some signs of stress or anxiety are: a furrowed brow, hands clasped together in a wringing fashion, or arms tightly clasped to the chest. The patient's legs may be crossed, or his feet or toes curled under tightly. The patient's head may be tilted back slightly, with the patient breathing in short gasping breaths.

The patient you are about to view in this audiovisual presentation is an asthmatic. Though the patient's primary complaint is one of lack of breath, the patients' evident signs of stress, discomfort and anxiety are universal to the majority of hospital patients. Once you have made a visual assessment of the patient, you may approach the bed and make the initial introduction. This first contact with the patient is extremely important and is the key to your future success with the patient. Always introduce yourself in a professional and caring manner. Let the patient know that you are there at the physician's request. And that the doctor feels the patient will benefit from your services. Explain that you are an experienced hypnotic operator, who specializes in helping patients experience increased comfort, rest, sleep and an overall sense of wellbeing while in the hospital.

While speaking with the patient, continue to observe their physical response to your presence. Note how receptive or how resistive the patient is to your presence. Ask if the patient has any questions about who you are and why you are there.

Always maintain direct eye contact with the patient and try to keep this eye contact as much as possible, because keeping direct eye contact helps the patient to maintain a point of focus away from his discomfort. Also, the patient's understanding of the information you are providing is greatly helped by maintaining direct eye contact. After you have explained the benefit of hypnosis, ask the patient if they would like to experience the benefits that you have mentioned. In the majority of cases, the patient will answer favorably.

Ask the patient to describe in their own words what their physical complaint is and how it is affecting them, especially in relation to sleep and comfort. The patient's own acknowledgement of their own stress or distress will give you insight into how you can best help them. In addition, it leaves the patient in a position of recognizing possible adverse symptoms in themselves. At this point, both of you can begin to set realistic goals in relation to your hypnotic services.

As a professional hypnotist, you have a variety of hypnotic induction techniques at your disposal. I have found after many years of using hypnosis in a hospital environment, that a rapid induction technique is the most effective. My favourite is rapid eye closure technique. Have the patient place his or her arms at their side, while placing their legs slightly apart. This will help to promote a deeper and faster hypnotic response. If the patient does not do this voluntarily, you can assist by physically placing the patient's arms and legs in the desired position. Now you are ready to hypnotize the patient.

In using rapid eye closure, bring your hand directly over the patient's forehead, telling them as you bring their hand down over their eyes, they will close their eyelids down. And they will leave them closed down. Next, bring your hand down, telling the patient to close his eyelids down as your hand passes over them. With the patient's eyes closed, tell them to imagine that they are a child, playing a pretend game and that this pretend game involves their eyelids remaining closed. And that their eyelids feel so heavy, so limp, so lazy and so relaxed that their only desire is to leave them closed down. Now count backward from 3 to 1. On the count of 1 snap your fingers and say "sleep now". At this point, you may assume that hypnosis has been induced. You can then condition the patient for future response, after which you are ready to work with the goal setting that you and the patient have agreed upon.

Before awakening the patient, it is most helpful to give them a trigger word and an image that will help them to experience these same pleasant sensations of trance when you are not there. Imagery is an effective tool in accomplishing this and strong post-hypnotic suggestions reinforcing the image make it far more effective. The imagery can be simple in detail.

Perhaps a scene from the outdoors, the mountains, or even the sea. You can always ask what the patient finds appealing. And what suggests to them comfort, peace and relaxation. For example, it would be foolish to suggest an image of flowers if the patient has allergic reaction to flowers. You should have some idea of which images you will introduce before your hypnotic induction. Always be aware of the patient's physical response to hypnosis, some of which are: the patient's brow smoothes out, arms and legs become limp and heavy. The patient's respiratory pattern may slow down. They may even develop deep involuntary breathing and their feet are likely to turn outward and the toes no longer curl under. The jaw may open slightly, the patient may exhibit one or more of these signs, though not necessarily within the same session.

With progressive hypnotic conditioning, the patient will respond with deeper and more profound physical and mental relaxation. When you're ready to awaken the patient, you need to reinforce the hypnotic response for your next contact with the patient. On awakening the patient, give him the choice of opening his eyelids immediately, as you direct him to, or of opening them when he is ready to open them. Because of the intense degree of relaxation, and the special quality of comfort that the patient is experiencing, sometimes they want to continue lying there with their eyes closed, just enjoying the sensations of well-being that they are experiencing.

In any case, continue with the trans-termination process, while telling the patient that when he decides to open his eyelids, he will feel just as comfortable and relaxed as he does with his eyes closed down. Always let the patient know when you're going to leave him, or if you're going to speak to the doctor or nurse in his presence, and if you're going to leave him, when you will return.

A valuable tool that you can use with the patient is the pre-recorded hypnosis relaxation cassette tape. This tape is an invaluable tool for helping reinforce post-hypnotic suggestions and for encouraging a relaxation response, at any time of the day or night that the patient may feel that they need it. You can introduce these programs to the patient in the same manner as you introduced your hypnotic services.

Again, it is important to set up patient expectation and realistic goals for both yourself as well as the patient. Explain the content of the program to the patient and ask the patient if they would prefer to listen to the program through a loudspeaker or through the use of headphones. If the patient decides to use headphones, be sure to provide lightweight comfortable headphones. Always ensure the patient's privacy by taking the phone off the hook and letting the nurse know the patient is using a cassette tape. Take time to observe the patient's initial response to the listening program. The patient after one or two uses should be able to use the program without your assistance, or perhaps with the assistance of the nurse. By helping the patient realize simple and easy goals in the beginning, the patient begins to develop self-confidence, overcome feelings of helplessness and develop feelings of personal accomplishment.

Remember to communicate your progress and goal setting to the patient's nurse or other appropriate healthcare provider. The techniques and procedures shown here have been tested for more than 5 years in a leading hospital and medical center in Santa Monica, California. They have, without exception, proven to be totally effective, completely safe and always self-rewarding to the patient, as well as to the therapist.

The hypnosis relaxation cassette program mentioned in this presentation is available from the producer of this film. The address is shown immediately following the copyright statement.

Gil: Welcome back, let us talk a little more with our respiratory therapist, John Silvas. John, why does the nurse, patient and hypnotist relationship need to be coordinated so carefully, what's the purpose of that?

John: Gil, the nurse is an invaluable link between you and the patient as far as ensuring proper delivery of your hypnotic services. The nurse can help you set up schedules, can help the patient set up expectations for your arrival. The nurse can also help reinforce your post-hypnotic suggestions. The nurse is your right arm in the hospital environment and I always encourage any hypnotist to communicate openly and frequently with the nurse as far as what they're doing with the patient , how they're doing it and when they will arrive and when they will depart.

Gil: Good. In the program we just saw you mentioned that you preferred to use the rapid induction process. Why?

John: Well Gil, in the hospital environment, time is very important and very valuable as far as money. So therefore, I had to use a technique that was not only rapid but instantaneous. And that's one of the reasons I studied with you, Gil. I found that you offered induction techniques that were instantaneous as well as being effective.

Gil: What is the purpose of the hypnosis relaxation cassette, John?

John: The pre-recorded hypnotic relaxation tape is another very valuable tool to use in the hospital environment. The reasons are, that it can be used when you're not present. It can be used any time of the day or night, and it can be used by the patient whether or not someone is in the room with them. It not only stimulates progressive relaxation, but it also reinforces your post-hypnotic suggestions, making the patient more receptive to future hypnotic encounters.

Gil: John, would you comment on developing the patient's mental expectation?

John: It is the most important part of the hypnotic process. In fact, Gil, usually before I meet a patient I will contact the patient's nurse and have the nurse, in advance, let the patient know that I will be arriving. The nurse, often times, will set up expectation by telling the patient that I am an experienced hypnotic operator and that I will be coming to help the patient experience increased rest, sleep, comfort and decreased physical and mental stress.

Gil: In other words the nurse, before you arrive, begins to sell the benefits.

John: That is right, she has already began the expectation process.

Gil: And then, the next day, you arrive.

John: That is correct.

Gil: And then…

John: And then at that point, I in turn begin to build on the expectation, helping to develop the patient's expectation of what they're to get. And I found that the patient wants relief and they want help, and that by expecting it from you and then in turn, you providing it, that you have a very mutual relationship.

Gil: Well this sounds as if a very special kind of bedside manner is an important professional quality in this relationship.

John: Absolutely, you have to present yourself in a professional, caring manner. By professional, I mean appropriate attire, either a tie or a related hospital coat, white coat, that symbolizes to the patient that you are part of the hospital system and you know what you are doing and you belong there. The caring part is showing the patient that you indeed care about their well-being and that in turn allows the patient to place more trust in your presence.

Gil: Wonderful. Well finally, in summing up, what would you say is the most important thing in supplying hypnosis services and benefits to patients in a hospital setting?

John: Well, there is two steps Gil. The first step is to find a school that trains you properly. That provides you with good background, good hypnotic techniques and application of those techniques. Secondly, you take those techniques out and you use them immediately. You go out there, and you do it, Gil. And by doing it, you become better and better.

Gil: In short, you were one of those who took the principle that I teach that the way to learn hypnosis is to start talking hypnotism after your training and to hypnotize anyone who will stand still, and for virtually any purpose that is a legal and ethical purpose for you to work toward.

John: That is correct.

Gil: John I want to thank you for being here. I know that you have contributed a great deal to people watching this program. And finally, in closing I want to talk of my excitement in being here with John. Because having trained almost 5000 persons in hypnotherapy, clinical applications of hypnotherapy, I am most excited by those who break new ground., who bring hypnosis into areas where it hasn't been used before. And certainly the hospital setting is one in which the safe, effective practice of hypnosis has been overlooked, largely overlooked. And the physicians and their applications of it, are one aspect of it, but patient care by other healthcare professionals such as John Silvas, Respiratory Therapist, and even more importantly, the nurse, because the nurse is in a natural position to use hypnosis effectively and to use hypnotic suggestion effectively.

Recently, our publishing arm, Westwood Publishing Company, released our latest book called "Hypnosis: New Tool in Nursing Practice" and we're convinced that this book, written by 12 nurses working in hospital settings, is going to revolutionize the practice of nursing, especially in relation to alternative healthcare practices.

This has been another production of Hypnos Production Company and we look forward to serving you with new and exciting training films in the future. Good day.

To Quote Ramtha:

"Love Yourself into the Future, and Watch the Magic Fall out of the Sky"

Transcript Of An Induction

An Induction I "Winged "and gave at the end of a HYP 203 course.

Alright, you are about to love yourself into the future.

So – there is a prerequisite about this. What do you really want to have the great pleasure to experience, enjoy, and sustain?

Make sure it is something for you.

Whatever it is – it is what you want to have, enjoy, experience, and sustain. It is something for you, knowing that everyone around you will benefit from it. The thing is: It is for you. You be alone in that picture.

So, as you are listening to the recording, it would be a good idea to write down what you want before you even start to listen to it.

And once you really know what you want to experience, to have, enjoy and sustain, take a deep breath – and as you exhale – close your eyes and become aware of your lungs. Your lungs – they are expanding and contracting, expanding and contracting, in a beautiful rhythmic manner.

And every breath that you take makes you go deeper and deeper into that really special quality of relaxation.

And as your breath flows, as it comes, as it goes, notice that the sensation is a little cooler, just a little cooler when you breathe in, than when you breathe out.

Just a little cooler, just a little cooler.

And let all your cares fade away, fade away, fade away, fade away.

As I am asking for your protection and your well-being and I say God, please allow only good things to come to you and for this blessing we give thanks.

And now you ask to be placed into the protection of your very own light, your very own light. Your spark of life. It is like a mini sun in your chest. Some people can feel it, some people can see it, and some people simply know it is there. That light of yours, that very beautiful light of yours.

Let it shine, let it shine, let it shine throughout every cell of your body, throughout your aura, cleansing your body, cleansing your aura, strengthening your body, strengthening your aura. Extending itself at one arm's length, above you, beneath you, at each side of you, in front of you and behind you and mentally repeat with me,

This is my body, this is my space, only light can come to me, only light can come from me, only my light can be here.

And as you take a slow deep breath and exhale, during this recording, as you are listening to it, the sounds of the room that you are in, makes you go deeper and deeper into relaxation. And during this experience, the music playing in the background makes you go deeper and deeper into relaxation.

And now, what you want to have, enjoy, experience and sustain – allow it to come into your mind now. You can describe it, and it is right in front of you – just cherish what you envision there, cherish it.
And as you are aware of it – that what you want to experience, enjoy and sustain – you take a deep breath, and as you inhale – bring it within you as though you want to swallow it. And as you exhale – love yourself into the future, and yes – watch the magic fall out of the sky.

That is right, what you envision there, what you want the great pleasure to have, experience, enjoy and sustain, it is right there in front of you.

Just breath it in as if you want to swallow it, bringing it into the now, and as you exhale – love yourself into the future and watch the magic fall out of the sky.

That is right, watch the magic fall out of the sky.

So do it again, it feels so good, it feels so great, yes, breath it in, as though you wanted to swallow it, bring it in within you. And as you exhale, love yourself into the future with joy, ease, grace, and gratitude. Your heart full of love.

As your subconscious mind is open and very receptive to the suggestions you are receiving now, it got the picture. It is shifts whatever has to be shifted, heals whatever has to be healed, improves whatever has to be improved, so that all this – or something even better – now manifests itself in your attitude, your behavior, your life – in a most delightful way.

And the benefits of this experience will stay with you for hours, days, weeks, months and years to come – much to your surprise and delight.

All this with great pleasure, joy, ease, grace, comfort and gratitude, your heart full of love. So enjoy it, enjoy it, love yourself into the future. And watch the magic fall out of the sky, that is right, love yourself into the future, and watch the magic fall out of the sky, your heart full of love.

(pause)

And when everything within you is in accord, everything is nicely synchronized and everything within you feels great, only then will you be able to open your eyes, feeling refreshed, relaxed, renewed, at peace with yourself and with the world around you. That is right, at peace with yourself and with the world around you, feeling great in every way.

Online Store, Contact, And More…

You may contact Anny by visiting any of her websites and scroll down the home page to the contact information.

http://www.annyslegten.com
Anny's private website and online store.

http://www.success-and-more.com
To find the description of the many services offered, and more.

http://www.htialberta.com
The Hypnotism Training Institute of Alberta including descriptions of hypnosis and hypnotherapy courses given.

http://www.reiki-canada.com
About the Reiki Training Centre of Canada.

http://www.slegtenianhypnosis.com
Although open to anyone interested in this fascinating hypnosis modality, this website information is for graduates of the Hypnotism Training Institute of Alberta.

http://www.connectwithanny.com
This is the best place to keep up to date with Anny – including seeing all her latest books and how to order them on Amazon.

Other Books By Anny Slegten…

REIKI PURE AND SIMPLE

Volume I: The Sacred Rites

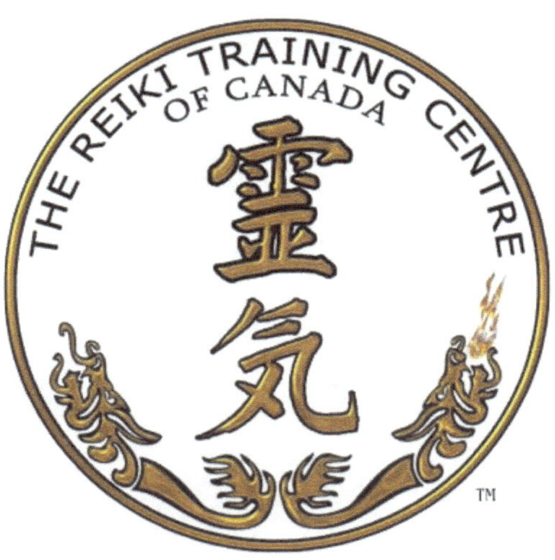

Anny J. Slegten

Reiki Training Centre of Canada
Class Material
http://www.reiki-canada.com

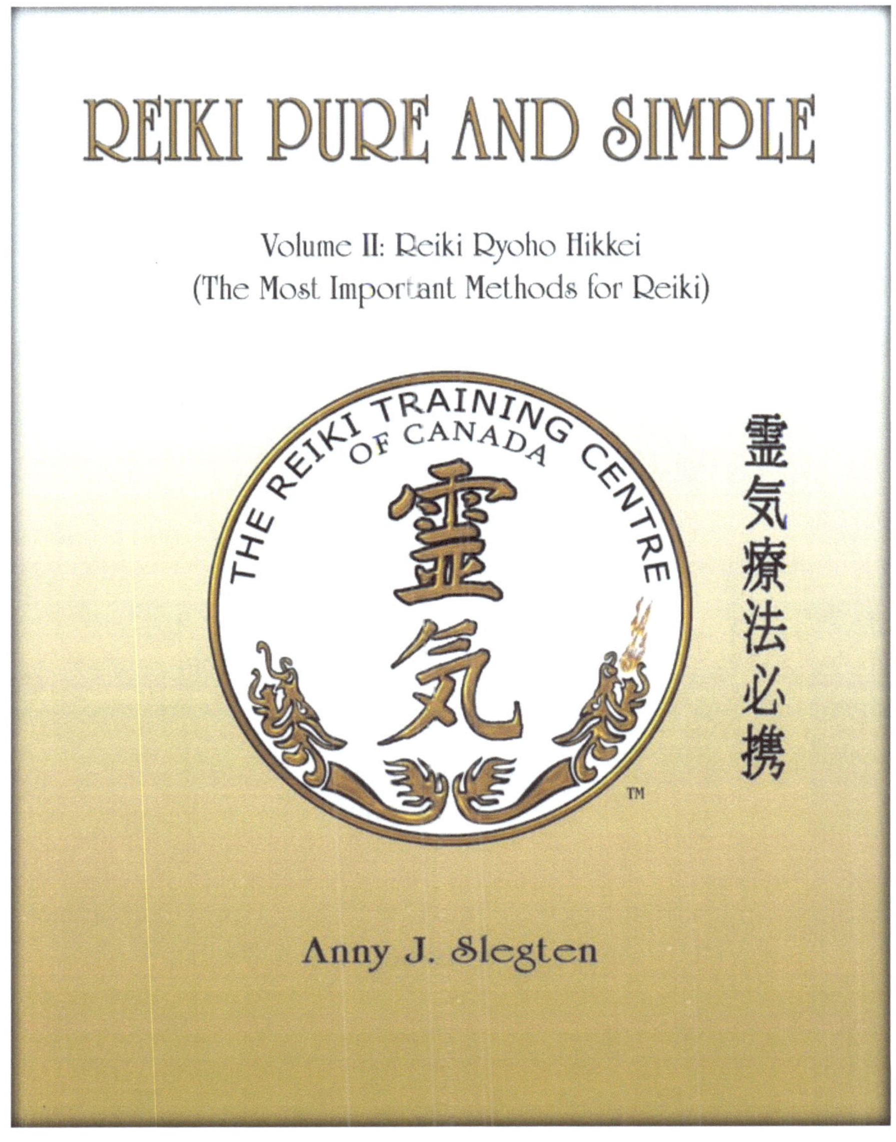

This book is a must read for Reiki Practitioners
regardless of their spiritual lineage
and could be of great benefit to Energy Healers
http://www.reiki-canada.com

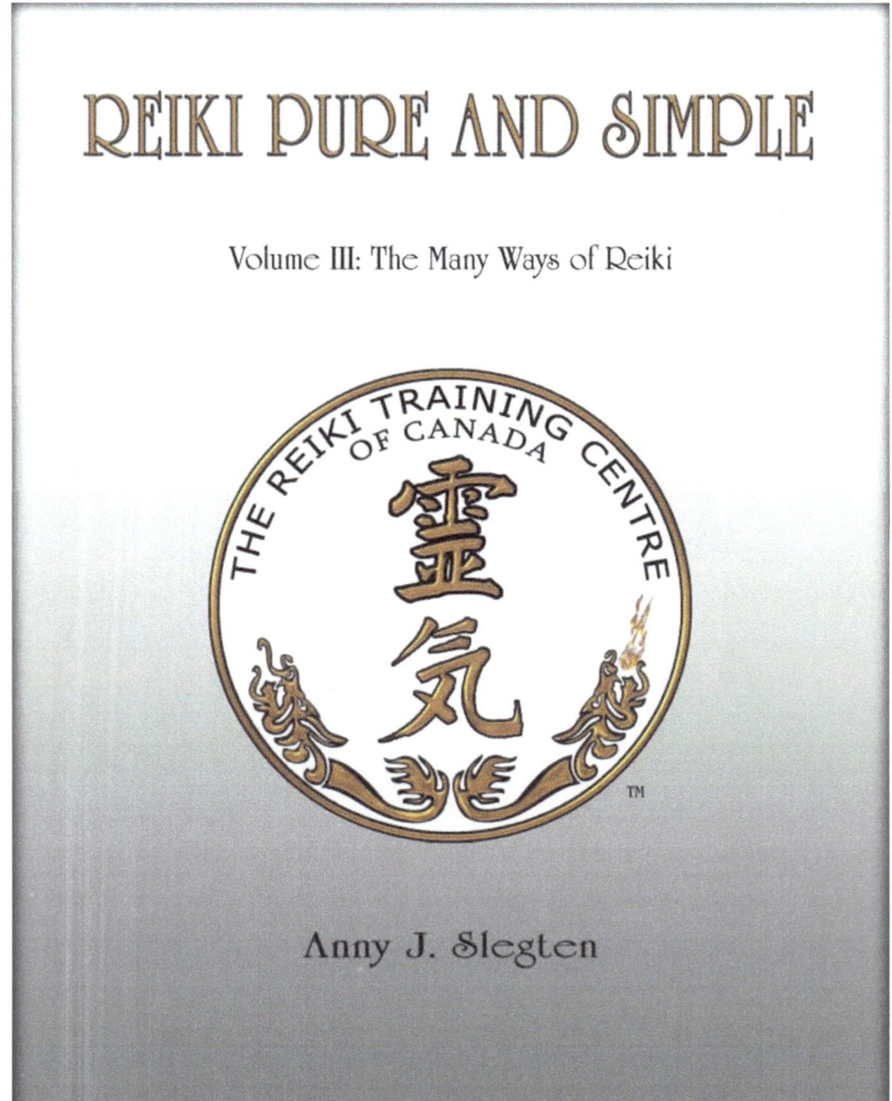

The Many Ways of Reiki
http://www.reiki-canada.com

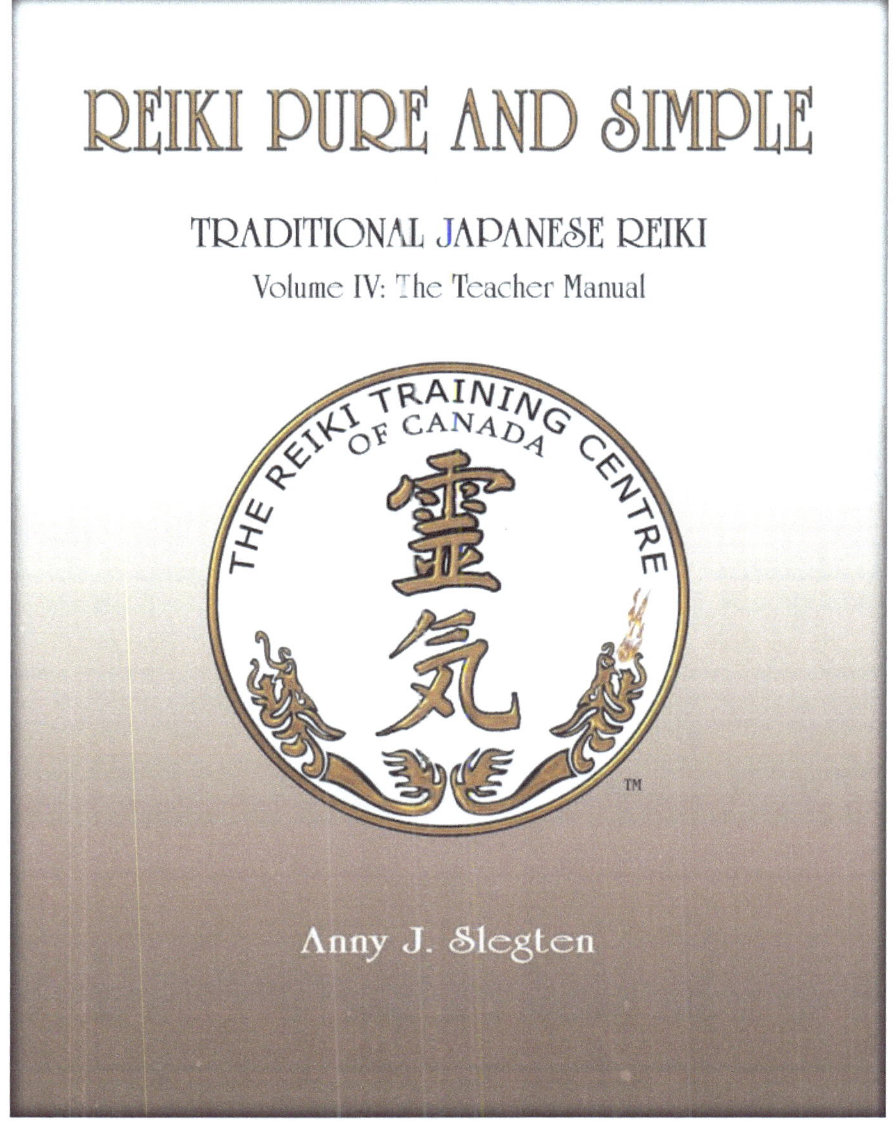

The Reiki Training Centre of Canada
Teacher's Manual
http://www.reiki-canada.com

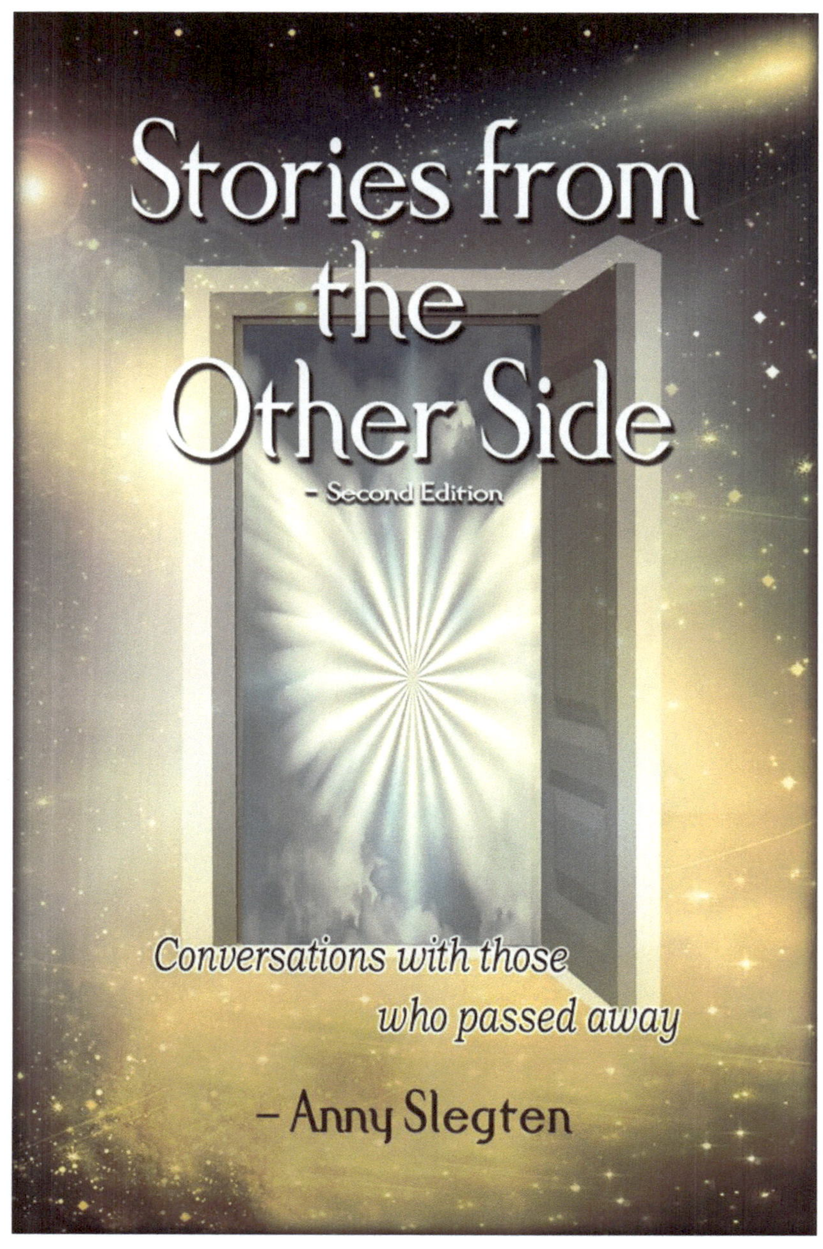

Stories from The Other Side – Second Edition
http://www.connectwithanny.com

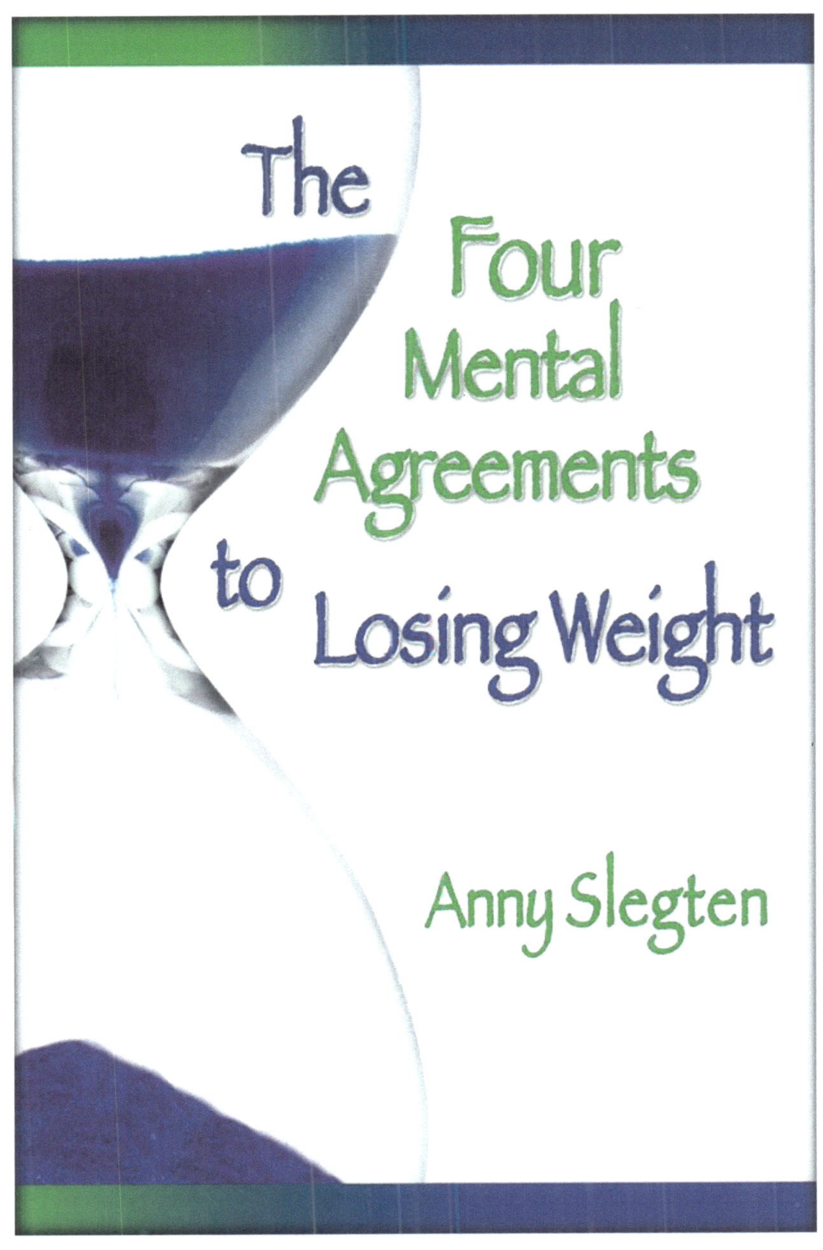

The Four Mental Agreements
To Losing Weight
http://www.connectwithanny.com

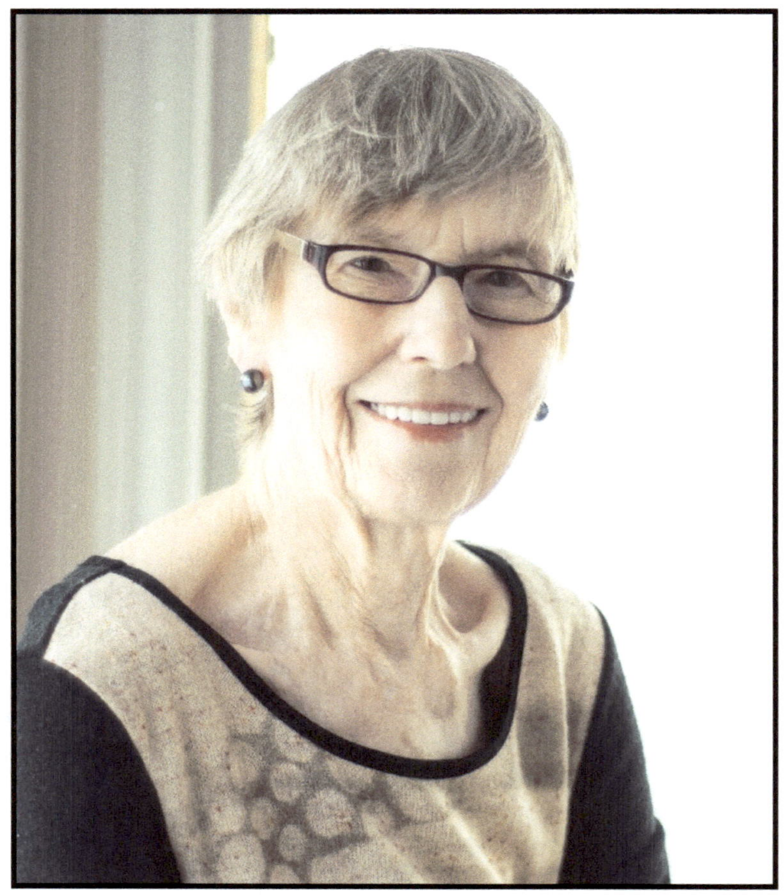

About The Author

As Director of The Hypnotism Training Institute of Alberta and The Reiki Training Centre of Canada, Anny has developed and structured the training and curriculum to the highest standards for both The Hypnotism Training Institute of Alberta and the Reiki Training Centre of Canada.

She offers training to students that come from all over Canada and around the world.

Anny has experienced and lived in many corners of the globe and this has given her a unique understanding of many cultures.

Anny's Belgian parents were from the Flemish part of Belgium and were speaking Flemish (Dutch) at home. Living in Congo, everything was in French.

Although she never spoke Flemish (Dutch), Anny speaks English with a guttural Dutch/German accent. Living in the English-speaking part of Canada for decades, Anny now speaks French with an English accent!

Anny is an Author and holds certifications as:

Master Hypnotist
Clinical Hypnotherapist
Hypno-Baby Birthing Facilitator and Instructor
HypnoBirthing ™ Fertility Therapist for Men & Women
Reiki Master/Teacher
Master Remote Viewer

Anny is a world renowned Clinical Hypnotherapist and Hypnologist in full time practice since 1984 as well as a Hypno-Energy worker since 2008.

In 1986 Anny created and developed an unique method using hypnosis for distance services - Virtual Sessions.

Over the years these Virtual Sessions proved to be an effective, useful, and efficient method for investigations and putting closure on both present and past issues - resulting in peace of mind.

To know more about Anny, please visit www.annyslegten.com and make sure to read what she published on her Blog.

Do you wonder what else Anny is publishing?

Visit www.connectwithanny.com

www.ingramcontent.com/pod-product-compliance
Lightning Source LLC
Chambersburg PA
CBHW050813220326
41598CB00006B/199
* 9 7 8 1 7 7 5 2 4 8 9 7 2 *